Bible Healing Study Course

Kenneth E. Hagin

22 21 20 19 18 17 16   18 17 16 15 14 13 12

Bible Healing Study Course
ISBN-13: 978-0-89276-086-2
ISBN-10: 0-89276-086-9

In the U.S. write:
Kenneth Hagin Ministries
P.O. Box 50126
Tulsa, OK 74150-0126
1-888-28-FAITH
rhema.org

In Canada write:
Kenneth Hagin Ministries of Canada
P.O. Box 335, Station D
Etobicoke (Toronto), Ontario
Canada M9A 4X3
1-866-70-RHEMA
rhemacanada.org

Contents

Chapter 1

Healing: God at Work

Some Christians who need healing have said to me, "Maybe God put this sickness on me for some purpose."

Did Jesus ever put sickness on anyone? When people came to Him for healing, did He ever turn even one away saying, "No, it's not My will. Just suffer a little longer. You're just not pious enough"?

No! Not once!

And the Scriptures tell us that to see God, we look at Jesus. Jesus Himself said:

JOHN 14:9,10
9 . . . Have I [Jesus] been so long time with you, and yet hast thou not known me, Philip? he that hath seen me hath seen the Father; and how sayest thou then, Shew us the Father?
10 Believest thou not that I am in the Father, and the Father in me? the words that I speak unto you I speak not of myself: but the Father that dwelleth in me, he doeth the works.

God at Work

Do you want to know what God is like? Look at Jesus. Do you want to see God at work? Look at Jesus. Do you want to know the will of God? Look at Jesus. Jesus is the will of God in action (John 6:38). Did Jesus go about making people sick? No! He went about doing good and healing!

ACTS 10:38
38 How God anointed Jesus of Nazareth with the Holy Ghost and with power: who went about doing good, and healing all that were oppressed of the devil. . . .

From the natural standpoint, it is difficult for people to understand that most of the laws governing this earth today came into being through the fall of man—when Adam sinned and the curse came upon the earth. Because people don't understand this, they accuse God of accidents, sickness, and the death of loved ones. And God is not the author of any of these things.

People also blame God for the storms, catastrophes, earthquakes, and floods that occur. Even insurance policies call these "acts of God." No, they are not acts of God. They are acts of the devil. Their author is Satan.

All of these natural laws as we understand them were set aside by Jesus, whenever necessary, in order to bless humanity. Bear in mind that Jesus said, "He that has seen Me has seen the Father" (John 14:9). Well, we don't see Jesus bringing any storms on people. We see Him *calming* the storms!

Rebuker of Storms

A storm had arisen on the Sea of Galilee and Jesus was in the back of the ship asleep on a pillow. The disciples awoke Him and said, "Master, carest Thou not that we perish?" They thought they were going down at sea. But Jesus arose and *rebuked* the wind. He wasn't rebuking something God did. He was rebuking something the devil had stirred up.

You see, Adam was originally the god, so to speak, of this world. God made the world and the fullness thereof (Ps. 89:11). Then He made man, Adam. He said to Adam, "I give you the authority to rule this earth. You are the one who dominates." But Adam sold us all out to the devil. (He didn't have the *moral* right to do it, but he had the *legal* right, because the earth was his—God put it into his hands.)

Adam committed high treason and sold out to the devil. And the Bible tells us that now Satan is the god of this world (2 Cor. 4:4). When did Satan become the god of this world? After Adam sinned.

Under Control?

We need to get some of these things straight in our minds, because many in the church world are confused. People have all kinds of unscriptural ideas. Some think, *Well, God's got everything under control.* But that may or may not be so, according to how you mean it. If you mean that God is ruling the earth right now—no, He isn't! He's going to rule it again one of these days, but He's not right now.

During the Korean conflict, I read an article by a well-known newspaper columnist. He said, in effect, "I don't claim to be a Christian, but I'm not an atheist or an agnostic. The atheist says there is no God. I believe there is one. The agnostic says there may be a God; he doesn't know. I believe there is.

"I don't believe everything just happened into being," he continued. "I believe some Supreme Being created everything. But what hinders me from being a Christian is what I hear preachers saying. I'm confused because they say God is running everything. And if He is, He sure has things in a mess."

Then the man alluded to wars, children being killed, poverty, disease, and sickness, saying, "I believe that there is a Supreme Being somewhere and that everything He made was beautiful and good. I just can't believe those things are the work of God."

Well, the truth is, those things came with the Fall when Adam sinned and Satan became the god of this world. When Satan is finally eliminated from the earth, there will be nothing that will hurt or destroy. And then it ought to be obvious where all those things came from.

Jesus' statement, "He that hath seen Me hath seen the Father," and His description of the Father make it impossible to accept the teaching that sickness and disease are from God. The very nature of God refutes such an idea, for God is love.

Let's go back to Acts 10:38 for a moment. Who anointed Jesus of Nazareth? God did! And Jesus said, "*. . . the Father that dwelleth in me, he doeth the works*" (John 14:10).

How did God do these works of healing through Jesus? By anointing Him with the Holy Ghost and with healing power. What did Jesus do with the anointing with which God had anointed Him? He went about doing good! What was the good that He did? Healing! So God was

healing when Jesus healed, because it was God who anointed Him.

God is in the healing business, not in the sickness business! God is in the delivering business, not in the bondage business!

Jesus Healed All

Notice in Acts 10:38 who was healed by Jesus: "*. . . ALL that were oppressed of the devil. . . .*" Now, that's a plain statement—all. *A-l-l!* That means everyone who was healed under the ministry of Jesus was oppressed of the devil. In other words, the devil had something to do with their sickness. That doesn't mean an evil spirit was always present. It just means the devil was behind the whole situation. They were oppressed of the devil—every one of them.

Yet to hear some people talk nowadays, even ministers, you would be led to believe that God and the devil had swapped jobs for the last 2,000 years! You'd think God was putting sickness on people and the devil was healing them. No, the devil is the same devil he always was. And God is still the same God.

MARK 16:15,17,18
15 And he [Jesus] said unto them, Go ye into all the world, and preach the gospel to every creature. . . .
17 And these signs shall follow them that believe; In my name shall they cast out devils. . . .
18 . . . they shall lay hands on the sick, and they shall recover.

Let's stop and analyze this. Which one of the sick did Jesus say to lay hands on? He just said *the sick*, period. Well, if God were the author of sickness, if He did put sickness and disease on people, and if it were His will for some to be sick, then this statement would be confusing—because Jesus authorized us to lay hands on *all* the sick and said they would recover.

If it were God's will for some to remain sick, Jesus would have had to have said something like, "Lay your hands on those whom it is the will of God to heal, and they shall recover. And those whom it *isn't* God's will to heal, they won't recover." But that wasn't the case. God set the Church against sickness, period!

JAMES 5:14,15

14 Is any sick among you? let him call for the elders of the church; and let them pray over him, anointing him with oil in the name of the Lord:

15 And the prayer of faith shall save the sick, and the Lord shall raise him up; and if he have committed sins, they shall be forgiven him.

Verse 14 asks, "Is *any* sick among you?" Among whom? The Church. So it must be God's will to heal any of the sick in the Church. Therefore, it can't be the will of God for "any" in the Church to stay sick.

Suffering With Jesus

"Brother Hagin," one individual said, "you've forgotten that the Bible said, 'If we suffer with Him, we'll reign with Him.'" No, I haven't forgotten. Let's look at that verse. *"If we SUFFER, we shall also reign with Him . . ."* (2 Tim. 2:12). Suffer what? Pneumonia? Cancer? Tuberculosis? No! What did Jesus suffer? Persecution! And you will too, if you live right.

You'll suffer persecution if you preach divine healing, the gifts of the Spirit, and faith. I've suffered persecution for preaching the Word in these areas. But I haven't suffered sickness and disease.

Another person said to me, "You've forgotten something else."

"What did I forget?" I asked.

"Why, in the Book of Hebrews it says, 'Whom the Lord loveth He chasteneth'" (Heb. 12:6).

No, I didn't forget. That's still in there. But it doesn't say whom the Lord loveth *He makes sick.* You see, people have just put their own interpretation on that verse.

The word "chasten" in the Greek means *to child train* or *to educate.* You train your children, don't you? And you send them to school to be educated. But have you ever told a teacher, "If my child doesn't do right, knock his eye out"? Have you ever said, "If he is disobedient, break his leg" or "Give him cancer"? No! That isn't the way you discipline or train a child. And that's not the way God does it.

Job's Problems

God doesn't use sickness and disease to teach His children a lesson.

"But God made *Job* sick," someone said.

No, He didn't. The devil did.

"Yes, but God gave the devil permission."

True, but God didn't *commission* it. You see, God will permit you to rob a gas station, but He won't *commission* you to do it.

No, the Bible is plain about why sickness came upon Job. Job had said, *". . . the thing which I greatly feared is come upon me, and that which I was afraid of is come unto me"* (Job 3:25). So he himself had opened the door to the devil by being afraid.

Bible scholars agree that the entire Book of Job took place in nine to eighteen months. And in chapter 42, you can read about the works of God! For example, Job 42:10 says that God turned Job's "captivity." That means when Job was sick, he was in captivity to the devil. When he was in poverty, he was in captivity to the devil.

But *God turned Job's captivity* and gave him twice as much as he had to begin with (v. 10)! Job lived 140 years after he got healed! That's God's work!

Paul's Thorn

Someone might say, "But, Brother Hagin, don't you remember that Paul was sick all his life?"

No, I don't remember that. And you don't either.

"But he had a thorn in the flesh."

Where did you ever read in the Bible that a thorn in the flesh is sickness? Nowhere. Go back to the Scriptures and see how that term is used. In the Old Testament, God said to Israel, "If you don't kill those Canaanites when you possess the land, they will be thorns in your side. They will torment you" (Num. 33:55; Joshua 23:13; Judges 2:3).

Paul tells exactly what the thorn was—the messenger of Satan sent to buffet him (2 Cor. 12:7).

Everywhere Paul went to preach, this evil spirit stirred up everything he could. He buffeted Paul in the flesh. And Paul couldn't command him to leave the earth, because he has a right to be here until Adam's lease runs out.

You can't separate sickness and disease from Satan. Disease came with the fall of man. The Fall was of the devil. Sickness and sin have the same origin—the devil.

Jesus' attitude toward sickness was an uncompromising warfare with Satan. His attitude toward sin and sickness was identical. He dealt with sickness the same way He dealt with demons. Since sickness and disease are of the devil, we must follow in the footsteps and attitude of Jesus and deal with disease as Jesus dealt with it.

Healing Is God's Provision

God always has been opposed to sickness, not in favor of it. Even in the Old Testament, He always made provision for His covenant people to be healed. If sickness was His will, He wouldn't have made that provision.

When Israel crossed the Red Sea and started toward their homeland, the Lord said:

EXODUS 15:26
26 . . . If thou wilt diligently hearken to the voice of the Lord thy God, and wilt do that which is right in his sight, and wilt give ear to his commandments, and keep all his statutes, I will put [literal Hebrew, "I will *permit*"] **none of these diseases upon thee, which I have brought** [permitted] **upon the Egyptians: for I am the Lord that healeth thee.**

Notice it isn't the Lord who made them sick. He said, "I am the Lord that *healeth* thee." God didn't put diseases upon Israel, nor upon the Egyptians. It is Satan, the god of this world, who makes man sick. Jehovah declares that He is Israel's Healer.

EXODUS 23:25,26
25 And ye shall serve the Lord your God, and he shall bless thy bread, and thy water; and I will take sickness away from the midst of thee.
26 There shall nothing cast their young, nor be barren, in thy land: the number of thy days I will fulfil.

As long as Israel walked in the Covenant, there was no sickness among them. There is no record of a premature death—no babies, young people, or middle-aged people dying. With sickness taken away from the midst of them, the children of Israel lived out their lives without disease. They just fell asleep. When the time came for them to go, they would lay hands on their children and pronounce blessings upon them. Then they would gather their feet up into bed, give up the ghost, and go home.

"What does that have to do with us?" someone asked. "That was back then."

Well, God is the same God now as He was then. The Bible says He doesn't change (Mal. 3:6). God was against sin in the Old Testament, and He is against sin in the New Testament. He was against sickness in the Old Testament, and He is against sickness in the New Testament. He made provision for healing in the Old Testament, and He made provision for healing in the New Testament.

Deuteronomy 7:13 says, *"And he* [God] *will love thee. . . ."* Love thee! Love thee! Love thee!

But some people must not be reading the same Bible. They read, "And He will put sickness upon you and cause some of you to be stillborn and some of you to die when you're babies and some of you to be sick and crippled all your life."

No! No! No! That's not the Holy Scriptures. Here is the Word of God:

DEUTERONOMY 7:13-15
13 And he will love thee, and bless thee, and multiply thee: he will also bless the fruit of thy womb, and the fruit of thy land, thy corn, and thy wine, and thine oil, the increase of thy kine, and the flocks of thy sheep, in the land which he sware unto thy fathers to give thee.
14 Thou shalt be blessed above all people: there shall not be male or female barren among you, or among your cattle.
15 And the Lord will take away from thee all sickness, and will put [permit] **none of the evil diseases of Egypt, which thou knowest, upon thee. . . .**

"But that promise is not for us today, Brother Hagin," someone said.

Are you sure? First Corinthians is in the New Testament, isn't it? Well, First Corinthians 10:11 says, *"Now all these things happened unto them [Israel] for ensamples [examples or types]: and they are written FOR OUR ADMONITION . . ."*!

Examples for Us

Glory! Deuteronomy 7:13-15 was written for my benefit! I think the Holy Spirit knew there would be those who would jump up and say, "That's just for the Jews. It's not for us!" So He wrote that what happened to them happened as examples to us. Those things "written aforetime," talking about the Old Covenant, were written for our learning (Rom. 15:4). Deuteronomy 7:13-15 was written for my admonition!

Do you think those people back then would be more blessed than the Church of the Lord Jesus Christ? Do you think they could be blessed financially and could prosper and be well, but the Church couldn't? Do you think that the Church—the Body of Christ, the Body of the Son of God, the Body of the Beloved—would have to struggle through life poverty-stricken, sick and afflicted, emaciated, and wasted away with starvation, singing, "Here I wander like a beggar through the heat and the cold"? No! That's not us!

We're Not Beggars

The Bible says we are joint-heirs with Christ, sons of God! We're not beggars! We're new creatures, blessed above all people!

You can see from the Scriptures that it was God's plan for everything connected with Israel to bear the stamp of prosperity and success. Disease and sickness were not to be tolerated among the Israelites, so the Church shouldn't tolerate sickness and disease either. Everything connected with the Body of Christ—the New Testament Church—should bear the stamp of prosperity, success, healing, surplus, and health.

What God said concerning Israel, He said in so many words concerning the Church. Romans 1:16 says, *"For I am not ashamed of the gospel of Christ: for it is the power of God unto salvation. . . ."*

I don't agree with all of Dr. Scofield's notes in his Reference Bible. But he was a Greek and Hebrew scholar, and his footnote on this verse in reference to the word "salvation" is excellent. Dr. Scofield says, "The Greek and Hebrew words translated salvation imply the ideas of deliverance, safety, preservation, healing, and health."

Glory to God! The Gospel of Jesus Christ is the power of God unto *deliverance*! The Gospel is the power of God unto *safety*! It is the power of God unto *preservation*! And it is the power of God unto *healing* and *health*!

God Was Israel's Healer

The Psalms were Israel's prayer and song book, and they continually mention that God was Israel's Healer. Psalm 103 is a classic example.

PSALM 103:3-5
3 Who [the Lord] forgiveth all thine iniquities; who healeth all thy diseases;
4 Who redeemeth thy life from destruction; who crowneth thee with lovingkindness and tender mercies;
5 Who satisfieth thy mouth with good things; so that thy youth is renewed like the eagle's.

Disease came to Israel through disobedience of the Law. So forgiveness for their disobedience meant healing of their diseases.

After God told Israel that the reason for their sickness and disease was that they had rebelled against His words and against the counsel of the Most High (Ps. 107:11), He said:

PSALM 107:17-20
17 Fools because of their transgression, and because of their iniquities, are afflicted.
18 Their soul abhorreth all manner of meat; and they draw near unto the gates of death.
19 Then they cry unto the Lord in their trouble, and he saveth them out of their distresses.
20 He sent his word, and healed them, and delivered them from their destructions.

You see, the children of Israel took themselves out from under the protection of their covenant by wrongdoing. Well, we have a New Covenant. The Bible says that it's better than the Old Covenant (Heb. 8:6). And we too have divine protection.

But it is possible to take ourselves out from under the protection of this covenant.

I'm not judging you. I'm judging me. I learned the truth years ago as a teenage boy on the bed of sickness. I was raised up after sixteen months of being bedfast: I was healed of two serious organic heart conditions, an incurable blood disease, and almost total paralysis. In the years following, the only time some physical disorder touched me was when I got out from under the protection—from under the cover. And, brother, I got back under it in a hurry!

When I say I got from under the cover, I don't mean that I stole something or told a lie on somebody. I just wasn't obeying God as I should. Perhaps He said to do something, or He told me to minister a certain way, and I went ahead and ministered the way I'd learned to minister instead of the way He said to minister. So I had to repent and get back in line. And the minute I did, I was immediately all right again physically.

For more than sixty-five years I haven't even had a headache. I've walked in health. And I'm not planning on being sick—I could be, but I'm planning on obeying God until I die. If Jesus tarries, I don't mind telling you that I'll live to a great age.

I'll know before I go, and I'll tell everyone good-bye before I leave. I'll look over on the other side and say, "There it is, folks!" And then I'll be gone! I want to leave everyone shouting and happy, because that's the way I'm going.

"But, Brother Hagin, you can't ever tell."

Oh, yes, you can tell. You can have exactly what God said you can have!

We have a better covenant than Israel had. If it was God's plan for the Israelites to live out their full length of time without sickness (who, by the way, were servants and not sons, under a covenant not as good as ours!), then imagine what His plan is for us, the sons of God! If God didn't want His servants sick, I don't believe He wants His sons to be sick.

I believe it is the plan of God that no believer should ever be sick. I believe every believer should live out his full length of time and, if Jesus tarries, actually wear out and then fall asleep in Him. It is not—and I state boldly, *not*—the will of God that we should suffer with cancer and other dreaded diseases which bring pain and anguish. No! It is God's will that we be healed. How do I know? Because healing is provided for us under the New Covenant.

Questions for Study

1. If you want to know what God is like, who should you look at?

    _____

    _____

2. Who is the author of storms, floods, earthquakes, and all other catastrophes?

    _____

    _____

3. When Satan is finally eliminated from the earth, what kinds of things won't exist anymore?

    _____

    _____

4. What two things make it impossible to accept the teaching that sickness and disease are from God?

    _____

    _____

5. What does the word "chasten" mean?

    _____

    _____

6. In Second Corinthians 12:7, what did Paul tell us his "thorn in the flesh" was?

    _____

    _____

7. For whose benefit was Deuteronomy 7:13-15 written?

    _____

    _____

8. What do the Greek and Hebrew words translated "salvation" imply?

    _____

    _____

9. How did the children of Israel take themselves out from under the protection of their covenant?

    _____

    _____

10. How do we know that it's God's will that we be healed?

    _____

    _____

Chapter 2

Healing: God's Will for You

In church meetings, I'm sure many of us have seen marvelous healings and miracles occur as the Spirit of God manifested Himself through the gifts of the Spirit. But I believe we sometimes think the only way God heals is through manifestations of the gifts of the Spirit.

According to First Corinthians 12:7-10, gifts of healings and the working of miracles are manifestations of the Spirit of God. However, we can't always guarantee that God is going to move spectacularly through the gifts of the Spirit, because the Bible says, *"But all these* [gifts] *worketh that one and the selfsame Spirit, dividing to every man severally AS HE WILL"* (v. 11). Therefore, we do not always know when God will move spectacularly through the gifts of the Spirit. However, we do know that God's Word *always* works.

The Word Works

We need to keep in mind that when the gifts of the Spirit are not in manifestation, people can still be healed through faith in God's Word. Therefore, we can always teach people the Word of God. In fact, I've seen just as many marvelous healings and miracles occur as a result of teaching people the Word of God, as I have when God moved miraculously through the gifts of the Spirit.

Healings and miracles can occur simply by teaching people the Word of God and by getting them to exercise their own faith for healing. You see, *the Word* is anointed. God's Word is the same whether I *feel* the anointing or not, and the Word always works!

Many times I think people are waiting for a manifestation of the Spirit of God to heal them. But they don't have to wait for a manifestation of the Spirit because the Word of God will always work for them!

For example, if doctors told you that you were going to die, would you just wait for a manifestation of the Spirit of God before you accepted the healing Jesus already provided for you? No, of course not!

Thank God, the Bible says, *". . . Himself* [Jesus] *took our infirmities, and bare our sicknesses"* and *". . . by whose stripes ye were healed"* (Matt. 8:17; 1 Peter 2:24)! If you *were healed* by Jesus' stripes, then you *are healed* now by His stripes.

I've seen more people healed in my ministry because they heard the Word and acted on their own faith than by any other way. Praise God, the Word works! That's the reason Paul told Timothy, *"Preach the word . . ."* (2 Tim. 4:2). Also, it's through *the Word* that we can be assured that it is God's will to heal us.

Satan Is the Author of Sickness

We know that it's God's will to heal His people because healing is in God's redemptive plan. We already read the scripture, *". . . Himself took our infirmities, and bare our sicknesses"* (Matt. 8:17). So we know that healing is in the redemption that Jesus provided for us.

We also know that it's God's will to heal His people because sickness and disease come from Satan, and God does not want us to have anything that comes from Satan. We really don't have any business with something that doesn't belong to us. Sickness and disease don't belong to us—they're of the devil. By the same token, healing *does* belong to us. Jesus purchased healing for us in the plan of redemption through His death, burial, and resurrection.

Unless our minds are renewed with the Word of God, we won't understand that Satan is the author of sickness, disease, and everything that destroys. Our thinking will be all wrong. But once our minds are renewed with the Word of God, we will be able to see that Jesus came to redeem us from Satan's power and to give us life more abundantly.

JOHN 10:10
10 The thief [devil] cometh not, but for to steal, and to kill, and to destroy: I am come that they might have life, and that they might have it more abundantly.

Jesus' Earthly Ministry

According to John 10:10, anything which kills or destroys is from the enemy. The Bible also plainly tells us that when Satan is finally eliminated from the earth, the law of sin and death will stop functioning: there will be nothing that will hurt or destroy (Isa. 65:25).

Jesus came to do the will of God and to set men free, not to hurt or destroy lives. Therefore, it doesn't make sense to say that *God* hurts or destroys people's lives.

Jesus healed people in His earthly ministry, taking sickness *from* people, not putting sickness *on* them. That makes it impossible to accept the teaching that sickness and disease come from God. Jesus plainly taught by His words and His actions that sickness and disease come from the enemy, Satan.

ACTS 10:38
38 How God anointed Jesus of Nazareth with the Holy Ghost and with power: who went about doing good, and healing all that were oppressed of the devil; for God was with him.

Be Loosed From Satan's Bondages

LUKE 13:11-16
11 And, behold, there was a woman which had a spirit of infirmity eighteen years, and was bowed together, and could in no wise lift up herself.
12 And when Jesus saw her, he called her to him, and said unto her, Woman, thou art loosed from thine infirmity.
13 And he laid his hands on her: and immediately she was made straight, and glorified God.
14 And the ruler of the synagogue answered with indignation, because that Jesus had healed on the sabbath day, and said unto the people, There are six days in which men ought to work: in them therefore come and be healed, and not on the sabbath day.
15 The Lord then answered him, and said, Thou hypocrite, doth not each one of you on the sabbath loose his ox or his ass from the stall, and lead him away to watering?

16 And ought not this woman, being a daughter of Abraham, whom Satan hath bound, lo, these eighteen years, be loosed from this bond on the sabbath day?

Verse 11 says this woman had a spirit of infirmity. Where did the spirit of infirmity come from? Notice the phrase in verse 16: ". . .whom *SATAN HATH BOUND*. . . ." In verse 16 Jesus also declared that this woman should *be loosed* from this infirmity and gave two good reasons why.

One reason was that Satan had bound her. We know that sickness and disease are bondages. God's people should not be bound by sickness or disease because Jesus already paid the price for our redemption in the New Covenant.

The second reason Jesus said the woman should be healed was that she was a daughter of Abraham. I've heard people say, "Yes, but that's Old Covenant." Well, we're under the New Covenant, and it's a *better* covenant established upon *better* promises. Certainly, if God's people can be healed under the Old Covenant, we can be healed under a new and better covenant!

To say that we have to be bound by Satan is wrong thinking! Galatians 3:29 says, ". . . *if ye be Christ's, then are ye Abraham's seed, and heirs according to the promise.*" And Galatians 3:7 says, "*Know ye therefore that they which are of faith, the same are the children of Abraham.*"

The woman in Luke 13 with the spirit of infirmity was a daughter or child of Abraham, and so are we—if we are in Christ! Jesus said this woman ought to be loosed. Well, if she ought to be loosed, then *we* ought to be loosed! Therefore, if Satan tries to bind us with sickness or disease, we don't have to accept that! We can be healed.

The Issue Is Settled

God calls sickness and disease satanic oppression. But, thank God, we read in Acts 10:38 that Jesus went about doing good in His earthly ministry, *healing all who were oppressed by the devil!* So many times people get confused and think God is the one who puts sickness and disease on them. But Acts 10:38 plainly states that Satan is the oppressor and that Jesus is the Deliverer! Let the Word of God—not man's ideas or opinions—settle this issue once and for all. *Healing is the will of God for you!*

EXODUS 23:25
25 And ye shall serve the Lord your God, and he shall bless thy bread, and thy water; and I will take sickness away from the midst of thee.

God told the children of Israel in Deuteronomy 28:15, "*. . . it shall come to pass, if thou wilt not hearken unto the voice of the Lord thy God, to observe to do all his commandments and his statutes which I command thee this day; that all these curses shall come upon thee, and overtake thee.*"

This verse doesn't mean that if the children of Israel disobeyed God, God would send curses upon them. It simply states that if they disobeyed God, the curses would *be able* to come upon them, because disobedience takes God's people out from under His protection!

By way of illustration, if you saw your child about to put his hand on a hot stove, you'd warn him, "Honey, don't do that! You'll get burned!" But if your child disobeyed you, and he put his hand on the stove anyway and burned himself, that wouldn't mean you *commissioned* or *authorized* that. Indirectly you permitted him to choose whether or not he would obey you, but you

warned him what would happen if he did touch the hot stove.

Well, it's the same way with God. And it's only in that sense that God permits certain things to happen in our lives, because He has already warned us in His Word about the consequences of disobedience. He said in essence, "If you walk in My statutes and keep My commandments, *then* I'll take sickness away from the midst of you, and the number of your days I will fulfill" (Exod. 23:25,26).

I've also heard people say, "I was sick and I learned a great lesson from it." Well, I'm sure that any child who has ever burned his hand on a hot stove learned a lesson too. He learned not to put his hand on a hot stove! But that wasn't the way his parents would have chosen to teach him. And sickness and disease are not God's way of teaching us either. That would be cruel, and God is not cruel.

The Word of God should settle the issue of God's willingness to heal you. Say it out loud: "Satan is the oppressor. Jesus is the Deliverer. With Jesus' stripes I am healed."

Jesus came that you might have life and have it more abundantly (John 10:10). Because God's Word declares that healing is in God's plan of redemption and that sickness and disease come from Satan, *not* God, you can know and be assured that healing is God's will for you!

Questions for Study

1. Why can't we always guarantee that God is going to move spectacularly through the gifts of the Spirit?

   _____

   _____

2. What do we need to keep in mind when the gifts of the Spirit are not in manifestation?

   _____

   _____

3. When the gifts of the Spirit are not in manifestation, how can healings and miracles occur?

   _____

   _____

4. People who need healing don't have to wait for a manifestation of the Spirit to be healed. Why?

   _____

   _____

5. List two reasons we know that it's God's will to heal.

   _____

   _____

6. What will happen once our minds are renewed with the Word of God?

   _____

   _____

7. In Luke 13:11-16, Jesus gave two reasons why the woman with the spirit of infirmity should be loosed. What are they?

   _____

   _____

8. What does God call sickness and disease?

   _____

   _____

9. Why do we know sickness and disease are not God's way of teaching us?

   _____

   _____

10. According to John 10:10, why did Jesus come?

    _____

    _____

Chapter 3

Two Streams of Healing

I've noticed that in the church world, people tend to treat important subjects like faith and prayer in a very general way. I think the same thing has happened with the subject of healing. Many times people just put all the scriptures on healing in the same sack, shake it up, and pour them all out together. It's no wonder that folks have become confused.

We need to learn to rightly divide the Word of God on every subject. For example, when we look at prayer, it's important to recognize there are different *kinds* of prayers. One kind of praying won't work where another kind of praying should, so it's necessary to find out what kind of prayer will work in each situation.

Well, when you study the subject of healing, you'll begin to see that there are two streams or methods of healing found in the Scripture.

JAMES 5:14-16
14 Is any sick among you? let him call for the elders of the church; and let them pray over him, anointing him with oil in the name of the Lord:
15 And the prayer of faith shall save the sick, and the Lord shall raise him up; and if he have committed sins, they shall be forgiven him.
16 Confess your faults one to another, and pray one for another that ye may be healed. The effectual fervent prayer of a righteous man availeth much.

MARK 5:25-30,34
25 And a certain woman, which had an issue of blood twelve years,
26 And had suffered many things of many physicians, and had spent all that she had, and was nothing bettered, but rather grew worse,
27 When she had heard of Jesus, came in the press behind, and touched his garment.
28 For she said, If I may touch but his clothes, I shall be whole.
29 And straightway the fountain of her blood was dried up; and she felt in her body that she was healed of that plague.
30 And Jesus, immediately knowing in himself that virtue [power, anointing] **had gone out of him, turned him about in the press. . . .**
34 And he said unto her, Daughter, thy faith hath made thee whole; go in peace, and be whole of thy plague.

In these scriptures we see these two streams of healing: one is *prayer*, and the other is *being ministered to under the anointing*. Both will bring you the same results, but you need to understand that there's a difference between the two.

The Stream of Prayer

We know it's thoroughly scriptural to pray for the sick. Mark 11:24 says, "*. . . What things soever ye desire, when ye PRAY, believe that ye receive them, and ye shall have them.*" That would include healing, wouldn't it? Otherwise the scripture would have said, "What things soever you desire *except* healing. . . ." No, Mark 11:23 and 24 includes all things—*whatsoever* you desire when you pray—as long as they're in line with God's Word!

These same two verses of Scripture brought me off the bed of sickness as a teenage boy. I had been bedfast for sixteen months with a deformed heart and an incurable blood disease. Five different medical doctors said I had to die because medical science couldn't do anything for me.

But something inside of me, the inward witness, said, "You don't have to die at this early age. You can be healed."

I began to meditate on Mark 11:23 and 24, because something inside of me told me I would find the answer for my healing there.

Now God may use some other passage of Scripture to lead you. You can't just lay some pattern down and say that's the way it's going to work with everybody. But with me, He used Mark 11:23 and 24. When I acted upon those verses, believing I received my healing when I prayed, I was healed!

The Prayer of Faith

You can be healed through prayer. In my case, I prayed the prayer of faith for myself. And you can do the same thing, because prayer is one stream of healing that's available to all of us!

On the other hand, you may not be in a position to pray. Your faith may not be at that level, or perhaps you haven't been taught along those lines. Then the Scripture also says, *"Is any sick among you? let him CALL FOR THE ELDERS of the church; and LET THEM PRAY over him. . . . And THE PRAYER OF FAITH SHALL SAVE THE SICK, and the Lord shall raise him up . . ."* (James 5:14,15).

I want to point out three things here that will be a blessing to you. First, the very fact that James asks the question, "Is any sick among you?" implies that there should not have been any sick among them.

Second, it proves that healing is for everyone. He didn't say, "Let them call for the elders of the church, and those whom it's God's will to heal will be healed, and those whom it's *not* God's will to be healed won't be healed." No, he said, "Is *any* sick among you?" So then, healing must be for "any" who are sick among us.

Then we also see that it's the prayer of faith that saves the sick. The same Greek word "sozo" translated *save* here is also translated *heal*. In other words, you could read it: "The prayer of faith shall *heal* the sick, and the Lord shall raise him up."

A person can pray in faith and receive healing for himself—the same way I did as a young boy when I was raised up from the bed of sickness by faith in Mark 11:23 and 24. A person can also call for the elders of the church and let them pray over him—and the prayer of faith shall save the sick (James 5:14,15)!

James 5:16 goes on to say that believers can pray for one another that they might be healed, because ". . . The earnest (heartfelt, continued) prayer of a righteous man makes tremendous power available [dynamic in its working]" (*Amp.*)!

As Christians, we need to get this revelation down on the inside of us. The Bible says our effectual, fervent prayers can cause God's healing power to be manifested!

The Stream of the Anointing

The other method or stream of healing mentioned is *being ministered to with a tangible anointing* (Mark 5:30). In other words, you don't have to pray for God's healing power because it's already present to minister to people.

This is the stream of healing power that Jesus flowed in here on earth. Jesus never had to specifically *pray* for the sick because He was already *anointed* to *minister* healing to them (Acts 10:38).

Don't misunderstand me. It's thoroughly scriptural to pray for the sick, and the Scriptures instruct you to do so. But, you see, there was no need for Jesus to pray for something He already had—the healing anointing!

Jesus said in John 14:12: *". . . He that believeth on me, the works that I do shall he do also; and greater works than these shall he do. . . ."*

Well, if we're going to do the works of Jesus in any measure, then it has to be with the same anointing. Therefore, we should learn something about how the anointing works.

Jesus used many methods of ministering healing, but the most prominent one seems to be the laying on of hands. You might say it was a point of contact through which the anointing could be transferred.

Also in connection with the laying on of hands, the Bible mentions two different times when people touched Jesus' clothes and they were healed (Matt. 14:35,36; Mark 5:30).

As we saw earlier in Mark 5:30, when the woman with the issue of blood touched Jesus' garment, *". . . Jesus, immediately knowing in himself that VIRTUE had gone out of him, turned him about in the press, and said, Who touched my clothes?"*

The Greek word translated "virtue" throughout the *King James Version* means *power*. What was the power that went out of Jesus? It was healing power. It was the power with which He was anointed.

ACTS 10:38

38 How God anointed Jesus of Nazareth with the Holy Ghost and with POWER: who went about doing good, and healing all that were oppressed of the devil; for God was with him.

We know that Jesus works the same today because Hebrews 13:8 says that Jesus is the same yesterday, today, and forever. So if in His physical body Jesus was anointed with the Holy Ghost to heal and do good *yesterday*, then He's doing the same thing *today* through His Body, the Church. Therefore, He is *still* healing people by the anointing or power of the Holy Spirit!

Where did Jesus' power come from? God anointed Him with it!

Someone said, "But Jesus is the Son of God. He was God manifested in the flesh!" Yes, but the Word of God tells us that when Jesus came into this world, He laid aside the use of His mighty power and glory (Phil. 2:6-8). *The Amplified Bible* says that He ". . . stripped Himself [of all privileges and rightful dignity], so as to assume the guise of a servant (slave), in that He became like men and was born a human being" (v. 7).

Think about that for a moment. At age twenty-one, Jesus didn't heal anybody or work any miracles, yet He was just as much the Son of God then as He was when He was thirty years old. But the Word tells us that the Son of God *laid aside* the use of His mighty power and glory.

It was only after the Holy Ghost descended upon Jesus and He was *anointed* that He began to minister in the power of the Spirit (Luke 4:1-14). No miracles of healing took place until He was *anointed.*

So you see, it's the anointing of the Holy Spirit that brings the power! And this stream or method of healing—healing ministered by the anointing or power of the Holy Spirit—is still available today.

Faith Gives Action to the Power

Now there's something you need to understand about this stream through which the healing anointing is ministered: There is a role that *you* play as a receiver!

You see, even though God has anointed people to minister healing to the sick, folks must understand that healing is by degree. Therefore, it is based upon two conditions: the degree of healing power administered and the degree of a person's faith to receive.

When healing is ministered with a tangible anointing, the power of God is present to heal, but the person has a part to play too. It's the person's faith that gives action to the healing power of God that's transmitted to him.

Remember Jesus said to the woman with the issue of blood: *". . . Daughter, THY FAITH hath made thee whole . . ."* (Mark 5:34)! Someone might say, "I thought it was the anointing that healed her." Well, yes, it was, but it was the woman's faith that gave the healing anointing *action.*

Thank God, there are several methods of healing available to us because God desires for us to be whole and well. Prayer and the ministering of the tangible healing anointing are two of them. And with proper understanding, we can learn to flow with the Spirit of God in these two streams. Then we can use our faith to give *action* to God's healing power in our lives. But the main thing God wants us to know is that He wants us well and free!

Questions for Study

1. What are two streams of healing found in Scripture?

    _____

    _____

2. Prayer is one stream of healing that's available to whom?

    _____

    _____

3. Give two possible reasons why you may not be in a position to pray.

    _____

    _____

4. According to James 5:15, what kind of prayer saves the sick?

    _____

    _____

5. What does the Bible say our effectual and fervent prayers can cause?

    _____

    _____

6. What seems to be the most prominent method of ministering healing that Jesus used?

    _____

    _____

7. How do we know that Jesus works the same today as He did in the New Testament?

    _____

    _____

8. What do you need to understand about the stream of healing through which the healing anointing is ministered?

    _____

    _____

9. Healing is by degree and is based on what two conditions?

    _____

    _____

10. What gives action to the healing power of God?

    _____

    _____

Chapter 4

You Can Receive If You Believe

In my many years of ministering healing, I've discovered that the number one hindrance to receiving healing—you could call it the number one *enemy* to healing—is not knowing that it *is* God's will to heal. This is usually the issue you have to deal with in order for people to be healed. You have to get them to see that it is God's will to heal them!

I've also found that there is one group of people who do not believe that healing is for us today at all. In fact, they're sure it is *not* God's will to heal.

Then there is another group of people who believe in healing, all right—but they are certain that God won't heal *them*! They think they've been too evil, mean, or unworthy. (The devil will always bring up something.)

But we must not be found in either of these classes. We must get in the "Bible class" and find out what the Word of God teaches about divine healing.

My wife and I pastored for about twelve years, and during those years we never buried a church member. I just kept working with them until they were healed! I found out from experience how to help people receive their healing. Of course, sometimes it took me six months to help some people receive their healing, but eventually they were healed.

As I said, the main obstacle is getting people to believe that it is God's will to heal—that He *wants* to heal—and that they should be healed because it is His will.

Believe You Receive When You Pray

Let me share with you a scriptural reason why it is God's will to heal you: God promised to grant the things you ask for in prayer—when you pray *believing that you receive*. Let's examine what Jesus said about this subject in Mark 11.

MARK 11:23,24
23 For verily I say unto you, That whosoever shall say unto this mountain, Be thou removed, and be thou cast into the sea; and shall not doubt in his heart, but shall believe that those things which he saith shall come to pass; he shall have whatsoever he saith.
24 Therefore I say unto you, What things soever ye desire, when ye pray. . . .

Notice verse 24 particularly. Jesus is talking about prayer here.

People who do not accept the Bible say, "Mark 11:24 isn't for everyone." In fact, I once heard a minister say, "Well, now, Mark 11:24 won't work for everyone."

I always respond to this argument with the question: "Is *prayer* for everyone? Or is it that some are supposed to pray and others are not?" You see, the subject in Mark 11 is *prayer*; it's not simply gaining the desire of your heart. Jesus tells you how to get "what things soever ye desire" through *prayer*, doesn't He?

How many should pray, then? Everyone. Well, if everyone should pray, then this verse belongs to everyone—because prayer belongs to everyone.

Let's look at verse 24 again: *"Therefore I say unto you, What things soever ye desire, when ye pray, believe that ye receive them, and ye shall have them."* The *King James Version* says, "when you pray, believe that you receive *them*, and you shall have *them*." This is talking about the things you desire.

For now, we'll just consider one desire—healing for your body—and insert it into this verse. Now it reads, "When you pray, believe that you receive healing."

"But there's no physical change yet," some will argue.

I know it. Jesus said, "And *then* you'll have it." *But first you must believe you receive healing!*

"But I'm not healed!"

People who say this have already missed it, bless their hearts. They're going by their *heads* instead of their *hearts*.

When you pray, you have to *believe* that you *receive* healing, and *then* you will *have* healing. *When* are you going to have healing? *After* you *believe* you receive it. When do you *believe* you receive healing? *Before* you have it!

"But that doesn't make sense," someone will complain. "That's not even common sense."

I know. It's way above common sense. Did you ever read Isaiah chapter 55, where God said, *"For as the heavens are higher than the earth, so are my ways higher than your ways, and my thoughts than your thoughts"* (v. 9)? This kind of thinking is as high above common sense as the heavens are above the earth!

If you're a faith person (if you walk by faith) and someone is critical of you, don't feel embarrassed. The problem is that they can't see what you see, because God's Word is so far above their sight.

"That faith business! I don't believe in that!" People who say this are confessing that they're not saved, because the Bible says, *"For by grace are ye saved through FAITH . . ."* (Eph. 2:8). Doesn't it say that? Certainly, it does.

When you pray, *believe* that you *receive* healing and you will *have* healing. That's the revelation I received years ago as I lay bedfast and almost totally paralyzed on the bed of sickness. But I discovered that Mark 11:24 belongs to me! I still have the Bible I owned during that time, and you can see where I wrote in red ink beside that verse, "This means me!"

'All' Includes Healing

Now the Bible states that in the mouth of two or three witnesses every word shall be established, so let's turn to Matthew 21 and see what Jesus said about believing:

MATTHEW 21:22
22 And all things, whatsoever ye shall ask in prayer, believing, ye shall receive.

How many things will you receive? All things except one? All things except healing? No, *all things*. If this promise did not include healing, then it would read "all things except one."

What if Jesus had said, "And all things, whatsoever ye shall ask in prayer, ye shall receive?" Then we'd automatically have it made, wouldn't we? Why did Jesus put that one little word— "believing"—in there? Because the promise won't work without it! Believing, believing, believing!

Believers Already Have Faith

Some say, "That's my trouble. I don't have any faith."

Why don't you get saved, then? *Saved people have faith.* That's who we are—saved people, believers.

Once during a crusade, a woman stopped me after a morning class and said, "Brother Hagin, I want you to pray for me."

I asked, "What for?"

She said, "I'm seventy-two years old, and I have high blood pressure and a severe heart condition. In fact, the doctors have just given up on me. They say I can't live much longer."

"Well, what do you want me to pray about?" I asked.

"I want you to pray that I'll have faith to be healed."

I said flatly, to get her attention, "Well, I'm not going to do it!"

It worked. She said, "You're not?"

"No, ma'am, I'm not."

"You're really not?"

"No, ma'am. I'm really not."

"Well!"

I saw I had gotten her attention, so I asked, "Aren't you a believer? Aren't you a child of God? Aren't you saved?"

"Oh, yes, yes! I'm a believer."

"Well," I said, "whoever heard of a believer who didn't believe? You've already believed for the biggest miracle there is. Believing for the New Birth and being made a new creature is the biggest miracle there is. If you've already believed for that, you can't believe for anything bigger than that!"

I continued, "Now suppose you had a grandson away at college, and you wrote him a letter every once in a while. Would you always add the postscript, 'Be sure not to forget to breathe'? No, you wouldn't remind him to breathe, because if he's already breathing, he's going to continue—and if he's not, all of your reminding won't help him!"

I explained, "You see, you are a believer—that's who you are. And all things whatsoever you ask in prayer *believing*, you shall receive. I lay hands on people because I believe."

She responded, "I'll be in the healing line tonight." And she was.

When I got to her, I said, "Well, I see you've come."

"Yes," she said, "and I'll be healed too! You just lay your hands on me." (You can see how she had changed since our conversation that morning.)

I laid my hand on her head and ministered healing to her, but I perceived that she didn't have the baptism of the Holy Spirit. (She was born again—born of the Spirit—but being filled with the Spirit is a different thing.)

I said, "You don't have the Holy Ghost."

She understood what I meant. "No," she said.

So I laid my hands on her head again and said, "Be filled with the Holy Ghost!" And instantly, without stammering or stuttering, she lifted both hands and began speaking in tongues fluently.

The point I'm making is, this woman already was a believer because she was born again. And once you're a born-again believer, all the promises in the Bible belong to you. This woman wanted me to pray that she would have faith to receive from God. But she had His promises all the time. She just didn't realize it.

There's an interesting sequel to this woman's story. Twenty-three years later, my wife and I were preaching in a nearby state, and after one of the night services, my wife asked me, "Wasn't that Sister So-and-so [this woman's daughter] in the service tonight?"

"Yes, it was" I said.

She had left the church before my wife was able to talk with her that night, but she was there the next morning, and Oretha and I were able to visit with her. We wondered if her mother was still alive. She was seventy-two years old when I prayed for her healing, and if she was still alive, that meant she would be ninety-five.

We asked, "Is your mother still alive?"

"Oh, yes."

"How is she?"

"She's in the best of health. Do you know, Brother and Sister Hagin, she's ninety-five now, and she only recently quit driving her car at night!"

I'm glad we didn't let her die at seventy-two when the doctors gave her up to die! Here she was at ninety-five, "still kicking," glory to God, and driving her own automobile! Why? Because she found out that when you pray, "all things" include healing: *All things*, whatsoever you ask in prayer, *believing*, you shall receive. And that's who she was—a believer. So she could receive!

Say this out loud: "I'm a believer." Well, it shouldn't be hard for you to *believe*, then, should it? Start believing that healing is God's will for you!

Healing Is a Good Gift

A key verse in the study of why it's God's will to heal is a familiar one found in Acts 10:38: *"How God anointed Jesus of Nazareth with the Holy Ghost and with power: who went about DOING GOOD, AND HEALING all that were oppressed of the devil; for God was with him."*

Some people say, "I don't know whether it's the will of God to heal me or not."

Jesus said, *". . . I came down from heaven, not to do mine own will, but the will of him that sent me"* (John 6:38). What did Jesus do here on earth? We read in Acts 10:38 that He went about *doing good and healing*. Since that is so, then doing good and healing *have* to be the will of God.

People sometimes get confused about the character of God because they believe something other than what the Bible says about Him. *But if you want to see God in action, look at Jesus!*

Jesus said, *". . . he that hath seen me hath seen the Father . . ."* (John 14:9).

Always remember that Jesus' actions reflected the will of God in action. And what did Jesus do? He went about *doing good and healing* all that were oppressed of the devil, for God was with Him. That means healing is *good*, doesn't it?

This can be summed up in the text, Matthew 7:11: *"If ye then, being evil, know how to give GOOD gifts* [we found out that healing is *good*] *unto your children, HOW MUCH MORE shall your Father which is in heaven give good things to them that ask him?"*

No Quick Fixes

Before studying something else in Matthew, let's look at three questions James asks:

JAMES 5:13-15
13 Is any among you afflicted? let him pray. Is any merry? let him sing psalms.
14 Is any sick among you? let him call for the elders of the church; and let them pray over him, anointing him with oil in the name of the Lord:
15 And the prayer of faith shall save the sick, and the Lord shall raise him up; and if he have committed sins, they shall be forgiven him.

Notice that James is talking about three different things here: Is any *afflicted*? Is any *merry*? Is any *sick*?

The Greek word translated "afflicted" means *to go through a test or trial* or *to be depressed or oppressed*. The word "afflicted" does not mean sick. Also notice that the individual who is afflicted is to do his own praying! So James is really saying, "Is anyone being tested? Is anyone going through a trial? Let him pray." Notice it doesn't say, "Let him get someone to pray for him." No, James said, "Let *him* pray." (Another person could never be as concerned about your problems as you are.)

People today are looking for a "quick fix." But God doesn't have any "quick fixes"! He's not putting on any 99-cent sales. And He doesn't have blessings priced two-for-a-quarter. I don't mean to be funny about this, but it's absolutely the truth. That's the reason James asked, "Is

any among you afflicted? Let *him* pray!" (Him who? The one who's afflicted—and that means "her" too.) Then James adds, "Is any merry? Let *him* sing."

Isn't it strange that when someone is afflicted, that person usually wants you to do the praying for him. However, when he's merry, he doesn't want you to sing for him—he wants to do the singing *himself*!

Many times people are looking for someone else to tell them what to do. But you can't be responsible for other people, and you can't tell them what to do.

If a person will just listen to the Bible, he'll *know* what to do. "What if he doesn't know what the Bible says?" you may ask. Then if he'll get alone with God, the Holy Spirit will speak to his spirit!

The Bible says, *"The spirit of man is the candle of the Lord, searching all the inward parts of the belly"* (Prov. 20:27). In other words, God will direct you through your spirit.

I know from experience that this works. People have come to me for advice, and I've said, "Well, let's pray." And we got down on our knees and prayed for as much as an hour. Afterwards, when I asked them what their problem was, they replied, "Oh, I already have the answer, bless God. I got it while we were praying." I never did have to counsel them.

Our Counselor

JOHN 14:16,17
16 And I [Jesus] will pray the Father, and he shall give you another Comforter, that he may abide with you for ever;
17 Even the Spirit of truth. . . .

The Greek word translated "Comforter" in verse 16 is *paraclete,* a word that has a sevenfold meaning: Comforter, Helper, Counselor, Advocate, Intercessor, Strengthener, and Standby. What more would you need?

That's why James said, "Is any afflicted? Is any going through a test? Is any in trouble? Let him pray?" Why? *Because when you're in prayer, the Holy Spirit, who is your built-in Counselor, will give you direction!*

Have you ever noticed how many times the Holy Spirit will take the Word and open it up to you while you're praying? Jesus promised His disciples that the Holy Spirit would bring His words to the remembrance of those who believe in Him.

Whatever God said in His Word, He said to us. It belongs to us. And the Holy Spirit will bring God's words to our attention while we're praying. But He can't bring them to our attention if we ignore Him and run to other people for help!

Don't misunderstand me—others ought to help us if they can. But if we do what the Bible says, it will solve our problems. We will get *permanent* help.

Well, what does the Bible say? It says, *"Is any among you afflicted? Let him pray."*

Do you need comfort? There's a *Comforter* on the inside of you—the Holy Spirit. Do you need help? The *Helper* is inside you. Do you need counsel? The *Counselor* is inside you. Do you need an advocate—one who pleads your case? The Holy Spirit is your *Advocate*. Do you need an intercessor? He'll help you intercede. Do you need strength and someone to stand by you? He's your *Strengthener*. He's your *Standby*. That means He's just standing by in case you need Him. He's there.

Now let's look at something else in James.

JAMES 5:14-16
14 Is any sick among you? let him call for the elders of the church; and let them pray over him, anointing him with oil in the name of the Lord:
15 And the prayer of faith shall save the sick, and the Lord shall raise him up; and if he have committed sins, they shall be forgiven him.
16 Confess your faults one to another, and pray one for another, that ye may be healed. The effectual fervent prayer of a righteous man availeth much.

Many years ago, the leading Greek scholar in the United States told me that verse 14 in the original Greek literally says, "Are any beyond doing anything for themselves? Let them call for the elders of the church."

There are many directions we could go here, but the point I'm making is based on verse 16: *". . . pray one for another, that ye may be healed. . . . "* Healing must be a good thing, because God wouldn't tell us to pray for something that wasn't good, would He? And if it's good, then healing must be the will of God—especially for Christians.

Would God tell you to pray for something that wasn't His will? That would be stupid, wouldn't it? And I don't believe God is stupid!

What Is a Good Gift?

MATTHEW 7:11
11 If ye then, being evil, know how to give good gifts unto your children, how much more [some of you need to say that to yourselves until you start shouting about "how much more"] **shall your Father which is in heaven give good things to them that ask him?**

From the standpoint of the Fatherhood of God, Matthew 7:11 says that God will give good things to us. But God told us to ask for them. And He said, "Pray one for another." So healing belongs to us. Say this out loud: "Healing belongs to me. God wants me well!"

Our Heavenly Father gives good things to them that ask Him. Well, what is good? Acts 10:38 tells us that Jesus went about doing good—and healing. Healing is good!

I want to ask you another question, since we're talking about healing: *Is sickness a good thing?* If it is, we ought to never want to get rid of it. We ought to want to keep it. But it's not a good thing to be sick and off work, to lose your job, to see your children go hungry, and to lose your automobile and home. (You could ask just anyone on the street about that, and they would know better!)

Likewise, *Is healing a good thing?* Well, if you're hurting, doesn't it feel good when the hurting stops? Yes, it is a good thing to be well and healthy, to be able to stay on the job, and to provide for your family. Anyone would know that's good, even from the natural standpoint.

Let's see what else the Bible says.

JAMES 1:17
17 Every good gift and every perfect gift is from above, and cometh down from the Father of lights, with whom is no variableness, neither shadow of turning.

The Heavenly Father never changes. He doesn't vary the least bit. And every good gift and every perfect gift is from above.

That means sickness and disease could not be *good* gifts, because sickness and disease don't come down from Heaven. It would be impossible—*because there's no sickness or disease up there!*

In what is commonly referred to as "The Lord's Prayer," the disciples are told to pray, "*. . . Thy will be done in earth, as it is in heaven*" (Matt. 6:10). Now if it is the will of God for His children to be sick on earth, then it has to be His will for them to be sick in Heaven. And we've already learned that they can't be sick in Heaven, because the Bible says there is no sickness there. If we are told to pray, "Thy will be done on earth, as it is in Heaven," then we are told to pray that there *not* be any sickness on earth. It is just that simple.

If sickness can't come from Heaven, then it could not be a good gift, according to the biblical definition. Yet I've actually heard ministers say, "Well, we don't know what's good for us—God does. And He sometimes puts sickness on people."

God certainly doesn't put sickness on people, because He doesn't have any! You can't give someone something that you don't have. So if there's no sickness in Heaven, where would God get it in order to put it on you? He'd have to steal it from the devil, and God's not a thief!

Every *good* gift and every *perfect* gift is from *above*. This must mean the *healing comes from Heaven*, because Jesus came from Heaven, and He Himself took our infirmities and bore our sicknesses (Matt. 8:17)! Start believing this today!

Questions for Study

1. What is the number one hindrance, or enemy, to receiving healing?

   _____

   _____

2. When you pray, you have to _____ that you _____ healing, and then you will _____ healing.

3. According to Matthew 21:22, how many things will you receive when you ask in prayer?

   _____

   _____

4. What kind of people have faith?

   _____

   _____

5. When do all the promises in the Bible belong to you?

   _____

   _____

6. Why do people sometimes get confused about the character of God?

   _____

   _____

7. What does the Greek word translated "afflicted" mean?

   _____

   _____

8. What is the sevenfold meaning of the word "paraclete"?

   _____

   _____

9. According to Matthew 7:11, what kind of things will God the Father give to us?

   _____

   _____

10. Our Heavenly Father gives good things to them that ask Him. According to Acts 10:38, what is good?

   _____

   _____

Chapter 5

Is It God's Will To Heal You?

Scripture reveals the *nature* of God to us. It also reveals the *attitude* of God toward sin, sickness, and disease. God's nature has not changed through the ages. Neither has His attitude changed toward sin, sickness, and disease.

You need to know this in order to understand divine healing. In fact, the first principal fact you should know about divine healing is: *It is God's will to heal you, because healing is in His redemptive plan.*

The Bible says that in the mouth of two or three witnesses every word shall be established (Matt. 18:16). Notice that the following texts from Isaiah, Matthew, and First Peter all agree that Jesus took our infirmities and bore our sicknesses.

ISAIAH 53:4,5
4 Surely he [Jesus] **hath borne our griefs** [sicknesses]**, and carried our sorrows** [diseases]**: yet we did esteem him stricken, smitten of God, and afflicted.**
5 But he was wounded for our transgressions, he was bruised for our iniquities: the chastisement of our peace was upon him; and with his stripes we are healed.

This passage of Scripture is taken from the *King James Version*. A good reference Bible will have a marginal note by the words "griefs" and "sorrows" (v. 4) to tell you that the Hebrew words are literally "sicknesses" and "diseases." Dr. Isaac Leeser's translation of *The Hebrew Bible*, a translation authorized for use by Orthodox Jews, reads: "Our *diseases* did he bear himself, and our *pains* he carried: while we indeed esteemed him stricken, smitten of God, and afflicted."

MATTHEW 8:17
17 That it might be fulfilled which was spoken by Esaias the prophet, saying, Himself took our infirmities, and bare our sicknesses.

This text is clearer yet. Matthew is quoting Isaiah. If you check the reference, you'll find that he is quoting Isaiah 53:4. I like to say it

this way: "Jesus took *my* infirmities and bare *my* sicknesses."

I read this verse for years before I understood what it was saying: Jesus actually—literally—took the cause of our sickness and disease. He took our infirmities and bare our sicknesses.

We know that Jesus was made to be sin for us (2 Cor. 5:21). The object of His sin-bearing was that we might be free from sin, and the object of His sickness-bearing was that we might be free from sickness. This truth is also reflected in First Peter 2:24:

1 PETER 2:24
24 Who his own self bare our sins in his own body on the tree, that we, being dead to sins, should live unto righteousness: by whose stripes ye were healed.

Thus, three witnesses—Isaiah, Matthew, and Peter—tell us not only that Jesus shed His blood for the remission of our sins but that with His stripes, we were healed. Some people do not believe this. I once read a commentary whose author said that "by whose stripes ye were healed" does not mean physical healing; it means spiritual healing. So according to the commentary, your *spirit* is healed by His stripes.

God, however, does not *heal* the spirit of the sinner. He *recreates* it and makes the person a new creature.

Jeremiah and Ezekiel, prophesying in the Old Testament, said, *"Behold, the days come, saith the Lord, that I will make a new covenant with the house of Israel. . . ."*; *". . . and I will put a new spirit within you; and I will take the stony heart out of their flesh, and will give them an heart of flesh"* (Jer. 31:31; Ezek. 11:19).

Those who believe that God heals man's spirit do not believe that man ever failed or sinned. Their unscriptural propaganda says that all of us have a spark of divinity that God needs to perfect. No! A sinner needs to be born again to become a new man—the new creature described in Second Corinthians 5:17: *"Therefore if any man be in Christ, he is a NEW CREATURE: old things are passed away; behold, all things are become new."* (The marginal note here says that he is a *"new creation."*)

When a person gets *healed*, however, old things do not pass away and become new—just the sickness passes away. The part that was diseased becomes new. (If I have a boil on my nose and that boil gets healed, I don't get a new nose. It's the same nose I always had. Just the diseased part is gone.)

Therefore, First Peter 2:24 does not mean spiritual healing; it means just what it said. As I read further from this gentleman's commentary, I thought, *If this means spiritual healing, then the Lord Himself didn't know it and He made a mistake.* I was recalling an incident that happened during a meeting I held in Oklahoma.

If *We Were,* Then *I Am!*

One of the seven cooperating churches was pastored by a couple I had known in Texas. They said, "We're going to bring a woman from our church for prayer one night, Brother Hagin. She's crippled and hasn't walked a step in four years. We've taken her to the best specialists in the state, and they all say she'll never walk again 'the longest day she lives.'"

Ordinarily I minister under the anointing. But on the night she came, I had ministered to so many people that by the time I got to her, I was exhausted. (The Lord is the same all the time, but I am not. Potentially, the anointing is present all the time, but in manifestation, it's not—and when I grow weary, it is difficult to yield to God.)

Since the anointing was no longer in manifestation by the time I got to this woman, I couldn't conscientiously minister to her as I normally would. Her pastors had brought her to the meeting from a distance, and what was I to do? Just send her away?

No, there was still a way to minister to her—because God's Word never fails! The *manifesta-* *tion* of the anointing may wane, disappear, and be gone. But the Word of God is anointed forever, and His words are Spirit and Life! Hallelujah!

So I sat down on the altar beside the woman, opened my Bible to First Peter 2:24, laid the Bible on her lap, and asked her to read it.

Then I asked her, "Is the word 'were' past tense, future tense, or present tense?"

A look of recognition flashed across her face like a neon light lighting up in the dark. "Why," she said, "it's past tense. And if we *were* healed, I *was* healed!" (That is believing in line with God's Word.)

I said, "Sister, will you do what I tell you to do?"

"Well," she said, "I will if it's easy."

I said, "It's the easiest thing you ever did in your life. Just lift up your hands and start praising God, because you *are* healed—not *going to be—are!*"

I wish you could have seen that crippled woman. She had no evidence of healing. She had not yet walked a step. But she lifted her hands, looked up, and as a smile broke across her face, she said, "Oh, dear Father God—*whooo!* I'm so glad I'm healed! Oh, Lord, You know how tired I got sitting around these last few years. I'm so glad I'm not helpless and I don't need to be waited on anymore." (You see, she was acting on the Word. That's what faith is.)

I stood and told the congregation, "Let's all lift our hands and praise God with her, because she is healed." (And yet, from all observation, she was still sitting on the altar, crippled.)

After we stopped, I turned to the woman and said, "Now, my sister, rise and walk in Jesus' Name!"

God and hundreds of people are my eternal witnesses that she instantly leaped to her feet, and she jumped, ran, and danced—just like the lame man who went into the Temple, walking, leaping, and praising God (Acts 3:8).

We all shouted and cried with her. Then someone went and told a lie about me! He said, "That fellow, Hagin, healed a crippled woman last night."

But I didn't have any more to do with it than you or anyone else could have. *Jesus healed that woman nearly 2,000 years ago, and she just found out about it that night!*

The point I am making is that although that so-called minister said, "First Peter 2:24 doesn't mean physical healing," it was the only verse I gave the crippled woman! I thought to myself, *If that verse means only spiritual healing, then God made a mistake. He should have healed her spiritually, not physically!*

Friends, First Peter 2:24 means just what it says, and it belongs to us now. Bless God, by Jesus' stripes we *were* healed!

Our Rights To Be Healed

Jesus not only redeemed us from sin, He redeemed us from sickness. So it *is* God's will to heal you. Never doubt it, because healing is in His redemptive plan.

Not only is healing in God's *redemptive plan*, but because Jesus sealed the New Covenant with His own blood, we also have a *legal right* to divine healing (Heb. 8:6; 12:24; 13:20)!

The New Covenant guarantees us the rights and privileges that Jesus secured for us, which include divine healing. In Mark 11:24 He said, "*. . . What things soever ye desire, when ye pray, believe that ye receive them, and ye shall have them.*" Therefore, we have a *prayerful right* to divine healing!

Then in Psalm 23, the psalmist talks about Jesus as our Redeemer, saying, "*Thou PREPAREST A TABLE BEFORE ME in the presence of mine enemies . . .*" (v. 5). Therefore healing is our *provisional right*—our Heavenly Father has prepared a table of provision for us, and it includes healing!

Incline Your Ear

The Master is calling you to take your place at the banqueting table and dine! He invites you to partake of divine healing and every other privilege that belongs to you in Christ! How? By inclining your ear to God's Word, because God's Word is His will.

Since God's Word is His will, you could say, "The Bible is God personally speaking to me."

Someone said, "Yes, I know what the Bible says about healing. But I don't believe it just that way."

Well, if you have that attitude, you are not inclining your ear to God's sayings—to His Word. Instead, you are inclining your ear to your own beliefs and opinions.

Some Christians don't incline their ears unto God's sayings because they always want to hear something *new* from the Word. When someone preaches or teaches on the subjects of faith and healing, they say, "Oh, I've heard all that before." But those folks aren't inclining their ears to God's sayings!

You see, the Word doesn't work for you because you *have inclined* your ear once or twice to God's sayings. No, "incline your ear" is present tense. That means it's an ongoing, continual action.

Proverbs 4:20 and 22 says, "*. . . INCLINE thine ear unto my sayings. . . . For they are life unto those that find them, and HEALTH* [medicine] *to all their flesh.*" Why should you incline your ear unto the Word of God? Because God's Word is *medicine.* It's a never-failing remedy for all your flesh, which includes everything that pertains to your life.

Questions for Study

1. What does Scripture reveal to us?

   _____

   _____

2. What is the first principal fact you should know about divine healing?

   _____

   _____

3. What three scripture texts all agree that Jesus took our infirmities and bore our sicknesses?

   _____

   _____

4. In the King James Version, Isaiah 53:4 has the words "griefs" and "sorrows." But how are these Hebrew words literally translated?

   _____

   _____

5. What does Matthew 8:17 say that Jesus actually—literally—did?

   _____

   _____

6. What was the object of Jesus' sin-bearing? His sickness-bearing?

   _____

   _____

7. God does not heal the spirit of a sinner. What does He do?

   _____

   _____

8. What does First Peter 2:24 mean?

   _____

   _____

9. Because Jesus sealed the New Covenant with His own blood, we have three rights to divine healing. Name these rights.

   _____

   _____

10. Why should you incline your ear unto the Word of God?

    _____

    _____

Chapter 6

God's Word: A Never-Failing Remedy

God wants us to understand the life and power that's in His Word. When God made the world, He created the earth, the sky, and the great expanse of this universe with *words.*

But God's *words* are a never-failing remedy for any situation or circumstance that might come your way in life, including sickness and disease. Proverbs 4:22 says God's words "*. . . are LIFE unto those that find them, and HEALTH to all their flesh.*"

PROVERBS 4:20-22
20 My son, attend to my words; incline thine ear unto my sayings.
21 Let them not depart from thine eyes; keep them in the midst of thine heart.
22 For they are life unto those that find them, and health to all their flesh.

JOHN 6:63
63 . . . the words that I [Jesus] **speak unto you, they are spirit, and they are life.**

God's words are full of life, health, and healing, and they act like medicine. In fact, the margin of my Bible reads, "My words are medicine." Medicine for what? *For all your flesh!*

Proverbs 4:20 says, "*. . . attend to my WORDS. . . .*" That means *give God's Word your undivided attention.* In other words, put God's Word *into your heart*, and put out of your heart everything that exalts itself against the Word.

The rest of verse 20 says, "*. . . incline thine ear unto my sayings.*" *That* means *take in God's Word through your ear gates,* or *open your ears to God's sayings.* If you're attending to God's Word and *opening* your ears to His sayings, you're *closing* your ears to other sayings, such as fear, doubt, and unbelief.

We are to look at God's Word as well as listen to God's Word. Proverbs 4:21 says, "*Let them not depart from thine eyes. . . .*" This scripture doesn't mean we are to be continuously looking at the Word so that we never do anything else. It means we are to always look to the Word of God instead of at the circumstances. In the good times and in the bad, we are to just keep looking at God's words—at His sayings.

There's power in God's Word! There's healing in His Word too. Notice Proverbs 4:22 again: "*For they* [God's words] *are life unto those that find them, and health to all their flesh.*" God's words are full of life, health, and healing!

The Children's Bread

The Word has a lot to say about divine healing. For instance, in Matthew 15:21-28 we read that healing is the children's bread.

MATTHEW 15:21-28
21 Then Jesus went thence, and departed into the coasts of Tyre and Sidon.
22 And, behold, a woman of Canaan came out of the same coasts, and cried unto him, saying, Have mercy on me, O Lord, thou son of David; my daughter is grievously vexed with a devil.
23 But he answered her not a word. And his disciples came and besought him, saying, Send her away; for she crieth after us.
24 But he answered and said, I am not sent but unto the lost sheep of the house of Israel.
25 Then came she and worshipped him, saying, Lord, help me.
26 But he answered and said, It is not meet to take the children's bread, and to cast it to dogs.
27 And she said, Truth, Lord: yet the dogs eat of the crumbs which fall from their master's table.
28 Then Jesus answered and said unto her, O woman, great is thy faith: be it unto thee even as thou wilt. And her daughter was made whole from that very hour.

Healing is the children's bread! These are Jesus' own words! You can incline your ear to the fact that healing is your bread, because Jesus said it. That means if you're born again, then you're God's child, and *healing belongs to you!* It would help you to say it out loud: "Healing belongs to me. It's my bread!"

Some of you need to incline your ear unto that and say it long enough for it to register on the inside of you, in your spirit. The Word won't work for you if it's just in your head. But when the Word gets on the inside of you—in your spirit—then results are forthcoming!

God's Medicine

Proverbs says, "*. . . incline thine ear unto my sayings. . . . For they are life unto those that find them, and health* [medicine] *to all their flesh*" (vv. 20,22). Since God's Word is medicine to all our flesh, we need to know how to take God's medicine, His Word, and appropriate it for the healing of our bodies.

We take God's medicine by doing what Proverbs 4:20 and 21 says to do: (1) *Attend* to God's Word; (2) *incline* our ears unto it; (3) *let it not depart* from our eyes; (4) *keep* it in the midst of our heart. All these instructions imply a continual, ongoing action, not something we do one time or every once in a while.

In the natural, suppose you had an illness last year, and your doctor prescribed a certain kind of medicine for you to take. Then suppose you got sick again this year with the same illness, and the doctor prescribed the same kind of medicine for you. You wouldn't tell him, "Oh, no, Doctor! I can't take that medicine. I took some of that *last* year!"

The dose you took *last year* isn't going to do you a bit of good if you need medicine again *this year*. It's the same way with God's Word. For example, God's Word won't benefit you if you have the attitude, *I've heard all that before*. No, in order for God's Word to do you any good, you have to stay with it. You have to keep taking God's medicine.

You see, the Bible says faith is the victory (1 John 5:4). And faith comes by hearing the Word of God, not by *having heard* it (Rom. 10:17)!

Great Faith

MATTHEW 8:5-10,13
5 And when Jesus was entered into Capernaum, there came unto him a centurion, beseeching him,
6 And saying, Lord, my servant lieth at home sick of the palsy, grievously tormented.
7 And Jesus saith unto him, I will come and heal him.

8 The centurion answered and said, Lord, I am not worthy that thou shouldest come under my roof: but speak the word only, and my servant shall be healed.
9 For I am a man under authority, having soldiers under me: and I say to this man, Go, and he goeth; and to another, Come, and he cometh; and to my servant, Do this, and he doeth it.
10 When Jesus heard it, he marvelled, and said to them that followed, Verily I say unto you, I have not found so great faith, no, not in Israel. . . .
13 And Jesus said unto the centurion, Go thy way; and as thou hast believed, so be it done unto thee. And his servant was healed in the selfsame hour.

Jesus called the centurion's faith *great faith*! What is great faith? The answer is found in verse 8. The centurion said to Jesus, "*Speak the word only*, and my servant will be healed." Great faith is simply faith in God's Word. It's taking God at His Word.

God wants us to have the same great faith that the centurion had. He wants us to have confidence in the authority of His Word. Because of the centurion's great faith, Jesus said unto him, "*. . . Go thy way; and as thou hast believed, so be it done unto thee . . .* " (v. 13). I believe Jesus is saying to each of us today: "Go your way, and as you have believed, so be it done unto you."

The Bible says God never changes (Mal. 3:6; Heb. 13:8). What He has done for anyone else, He will do for you, if you will believe Him and take Him at His Word. God is no respecter of persons (Acts 10:34). He doesn't favor one person more than another. He favors anyone who is committed to believing His Word.

God's Willingness To Heal

MATTHEW 8:1-3
1 When he [Jesus] was come down from the mountain, great multitudes followed him.
2 And, behold, there came a leper and worshipped him, saying, Lord, if thou wilt, thou canst make me clean.
3 And Jesus put forth his hand, and touched him, saying, I will; be thou clean. And immediately his leprosy was cleansed.

MATTHEW 8:14-17
14 And when Jesus was come into Peter's house, he saw his wife's mother laid, and sick of a fever.

15 And he touched her hand, and the fever left her: and she arose, and ministered unto them.
16 When the even was come, they brought unto him many that were possessed with devils: and he cast out the spirits with his word, and healed all that were sick:
17 That it might be fulfilled which was spoken by Esaias the prophet, saying, Himself took our infirmities, and bare our sicknesses.

There are a lot of truths we could expound on in these verses. But I think one great truth that outshines the rest is God's willingness to heal everyone. Notice in the first passage that the leper believed Jesus *could* heal him, but he questioned whether or not Jesus *would* heal him. The leper said, "*. . . Lord, IF THOU WILT, thou canst make me clean*" (v. 2). Jesus settled the issue once and for all when He plainly answered the man, "I will" (v. 3). Yet many folks today follow the leper's *unbelief* about healing rather than Jesus' *willingness* to heal.

Now take a look at the second passage of Scripture from Matthew 8. In verses 14 and 15 we read that Jesus healed Peter's mother-in-law.

Many believe it is God's will to heal *some people* or a selected few, such as the mother-in-law of one of Jesus' disciples. But they don't believe it's God's will to heal everyone.

But notice that the same day Jesus healed Peter's mother-in-law, He also healed all those in need: "*When the even was come, they brought unto him MANY that were possessed with devils: and he cast out the spirits with his word, and healed ALL that were sick*" (v. 16).

Why did Jesus heal the multitudes? The very next verse says He healed them "*That it might be fulfilled which was spoken by Esaias the prophet, saying, Himself took our infirmities, and bare our sicknesses*" (v. 17). Jesus was moved by compassion to heal the sick (Matt. 9:36).

So we know from the Word that healing does not belong to just a selected few. God doesn't favor some but not others. For example, the Bible doesn't say, "Himself took *Peter's mother-in-law's* infirmities and bore *her* sicknesses"! And it doesn't say, "Himself took *the centurion's servant's* infirmities and bore *his* sicknesses"!

No, the Bible says, "*. . . Himself took OUR infirmities, and bare OUR sicknesses*" (Matt. 8:17)! And it was on the basis of this truth that Jesus healed the multitudes. Jesus healed "*all that were sick*" who came to Him (v. 16).

I've been in the healing ministry for quite some time now, and I have found that the biggest difficulty to getting people healed is to convince them that it is God's *will* to heal. Many Christians make some effort to approach God and receive healing, yet many times the thought lurks in the back of their minds, *I know God does heal people, but it might not be His will to heal me.*

But, you see, these folks aren't inclining their ears unto God's sayings. When you incline your ear to what God says, you *know* the will of God concerning healing. And over and over again, God's willingness to heal is expressed in the pages of His Word.

Let's listen to God's Word continually and incline our ears unto *His* sayings. I've said many times that just because I ate one T-bone steak doesn't mean I'm never going to eat another one. In a similar sense, just as continually feeding your *body* with good food keeps it strong, continually feeding your spirit with God's Word keeps your *spirit* strong and your faith alive.

When you feed your spirit on God's Word along the lines of healing, you are building health and healing into your body, because God's Word is health to all your flesh!

God's Word Is His Will

We can know the will of God in the situations and circumstances of life by inclining our ears to God's sayings (Prov. 4:20)! God's *Word* is God's *will.*

There is peace and comfort in knowing the will of God. As the psalmist of old said, "*How precious also are thy thoughts unto me, O God! how great is the sum of them!*" (Ps. 139:17).

In a few earlier chapters, we learned that Jesus' earthly ministry was the will of God in action on the behalf of mankind. Jesus said in

John 6:38, "*. . . I came down from heaven, not to do mine own will, but the will of him that sent me.*"

ACTS 10:38
38 How God anointed Jesus of Nazareth with the Holy Ghost and with power: who went about doing good, and healing all that were oppressed of the devil; for God was with him.

Was Jesus doing God's will when He went about doing good and healing all who were oppressed by the devil? Certainly, He was!

God Never Changes!

Has God's will changed about healing all those who are oppressed by the devil? Of course not, because the Bible says God never changes (Mal. 3:6; Heb. 13:8). So we can know for certain that it is God's will to heal everyone.

Acts 10:38 should be enough to convince us that it is God's will to heal today, but there are many other verses that also reveal to us God's will concerning healing. That's why we should incline our ears to God's Word—to His sayings—because His words are life to those who find them and health to all their flesh (Prov. 4:22). God's Word is medicine!

I've said before that the Bible is God speaking to each one of us personally, and that Jesus' earthly ministry was the express will of God in action. Since Jesus was God who came in the flesh (John 1:1,14), we could also say that *Jesus is God speaking to us personally.*

HEBREWS 1:1,2
1   God, who at sundry times and in divers manners spake in time past unto the fathers by the prophets,
2   Hath in these last days spoken unto us by his Son, whom he hath appointed heir of all things, by whom also he made the worlds.

If Jesus is God speaking to us, what is God saying? Is God saying it is not His will to heal or that it is His will to heal only a few? Certainly not. *God reveals in His Word that He never changes.* In other words, whatever He has done

for anyone else, He will do for each of us, if we will take Him at His Word and trust Him.

Are You Limiting God?

In His Word, God also reveals to us that He is a kind, loving Heavenly Father.

MATTHEW 7:7-11
7   Ask, and it shall be given you; seek, and ye shall find; knock, and it shall be opened unto you:
8   For every one that asketh receiveth; and he that seeketh findeth; and to him that knocketh it shall be opened.
9   Or what man is there of you, whom if his son ask bread, will he give him a stone?
10 Or if he ask a fish, will he give him a serpent?
11 If ye then, being evil, know how to give good gifts unto your children, how much more shall your Father which is in heaven give good things to them that ask him?

How much more will God give good things to us! This passage of Scripture is saying that as a natural father loves his children and desires the best for them, our Heavenly Father loves His children *much more* and desires to give us good things in life.

For instance, if your child was burning up with fever, how many of you parents would heal him if you could? Certainly you would make your child well if it were in your power to do so. Well, thank God, God wants to do the same for His children, and *God is able!*

Someone asked, "If God is able, then why doesn't He just heal every sick person?"

God is omnipotent or all-powerful. But He can only do in a person's life what that person allows Him to do.

Some will argue that since God is omnipotent, He can make people do anything He wants them to do. But if that were true, He'd make all sinners get saved, and He'd make all Christians pay their tithes!

No, God can't do any more in your life than you permit Him to do. Jesus said, "*Behold, I stand at the door, and knock: if any man* [will] *hear my voice, and open the door, I will come in to him, and will sup with him, and he with me"* (Rev. 3:20).

Man is a free moral agent—he has the ability and the right to make his own choices. He can choose to accept Jesus Christ as Savior and Lord and be born again, or he can reject Jesus.

Even after you are born again, you don't lose your will or right to choose. You have a choice as to what you will do with God's Word. Will you attend to it? Will you incline your ear to it? Will you keep it before your eyes and in the midst of your heart?

If you do, God's Word will become life and health to you. God's Word is a never-failing remedy for all your flesh and for all the problems of life that may try to come your way!

People bring a lot of trouble on themselves. And, of course, the devil accommodates them in wrongdoing too. People get into trouble when they don't do what the Bible says to do.

You can spare yourself a lot of misery in life by just doing what the Bible says—by inclining your ear to God's sayings!

Inclining Our Ears

You need to incline your ear to what God's Word says about every area of your life. When you obey one part of the Bible, it makes it a whole lot easier to obey other parts of the Bible.

On the other hand, if you disobey God's Word along one particular line, it makes it easier to disobey God's Word in other areas. And when you're in disobedience, it opens the door for the devil to try to work in your life. It's just better to listen and pay attention to what the Bible says.

We need to incline our ears to all of God's Word and let it be the final authority in our lives. God's Word is God Himself speaking to us. And the Word plainly reveals God's will, including His will to heal sickness and disease.

Some people read God's Word and still miss the fact that Jesus is the Healer. They ask, "If Jesus is the Healer and the Word is life and health to all our flesh, where do sickness and disease come from?" They think that if they're sick, *God* must have put sickness on them because He's trying to teach them something.

But if you'll get into the Word, the Holy Ghost will illuminate your mind and your spirit, and you will see that God is the Healer. Satan is the defiler—the one who tries to hurt people with sickness and disease. Satan is the author of sickness and disease, not God.

JOHN 10:10
10 The thief cometh not, but for to steal, and to kill, and to destroy: I am come that they might have life, and that they might have it more abundantly.

Remember, the Bible says that Satan is the thief that steals, kills, and destroys. And when Satan is finally eliminated from the earth—from all human contact—there will be nothing that will hurt or destroy (Isa. 65:25). So we know that anything that hurts or destroys is of Satan, not God. Sickness hurts and destroys, but God *heals* sickness. He doesn't *put* sickness *on* people.

I've seen people get attacked by sickness and disease and say, "Well, God must have put this on me for some purpose. He probably has some great, mystical purpose in mind." Bless their darling hearts. But folks who believe this way are playing right into the devil's hands. They are being robbed of the blessings of healing and health that God wants them to enjoy.

It stands to reason that healing must be God's will or He wouldn't have given us instructions in Proverbs 4:20-22 to tell us how to experience life and health in our bodies.

People who don't believe it is God's will to heal have a distorted mental picture of the character of God. And the only way they can remedy that is to incline their ears to God's Word. If they would listen to what the Word says, they'd get the right picture of God in their hearts and minds, and their spiritual viewpoint wouldn't be distorted.

Light and Life

PROVERBS 4:20-22
20 My son, attend to my words; incline thine ear unto my sayings.

21 Let them not depart from thine eyes; keep them in the midst of thine heart.
22 For they are life unto those that find them, and health to all their flesh.

I get more thrilled teaching healing from Proverbs 4:20-22 than I do from any other standpoint, because this is the way I was healed and raised up from a deathbed as a teenager. I had a deformed heart and an incurable blood disease from birth. I never ran and played as a child like the other little children did. I used to just sit inside and watch from the window in awe as other children ran and laughed and played outside. I didn't have a normal childhood.

I know what it's like to have no hope for a better tomorrow. Five medical doctors told me I had to die because medical science couldn't do a thing for me. And I know what people who are dealing with sickness and disease in their bodies are going through, because I've experienced that too.

While sickness and disease ravaged my body, I would just stare at the ceiling hour after hour, day after day, wishing more than anything else just to be able to live. I agonized as I searched my mind for answers. I knew there had to be an answer somewhere.

I remember those days when the sun was shining brightly outside, but the room where I was imprisoned by sickness and disease seemed to be filled with darkness and death. Gloom hung like a shadow over me as I lay there on my sickbed and planned my own funeral. I was only a teenager. I hadn't even begun to live, yet medical science said I had to die.

But, glory to God, I also remember when the light of God's Word came shining in! The psalmist said, *"The entrance of thy words giveth LIGHT; it giveth understanding unto the simple"* (Ps. 119:130). I couldn't even understand the Bible, but I kept reading it because I knew my answer was somewhere in God's Word.

MARK 11:24
24 Therefore I [Jesus] say unto you, What things soever ye desire, when ye pray, believe that ye receive them, and ye shall have them.

I had read Mark 11:24 before, but I didn't know what it meant or how to act on it. In the nighttime as I lay dying, I would repeat that verse over and over again all night long. I did that thousands of times.

At first Mark 11:24 was just words to me, but some way or another I knew there was healing for me in that verse. Finally, the light shone through, and the truth of God's Word dawned on my heart. I received healing from the top of my head to the soles of my feet. I got up off that bed of sickness completely well—and I've been well ever since!

"Yes, Brother Hagin," someone said, "that happened because God called you to preach."

But Mark 11:24 didn't work for me because God called me to preach. It worked for me because I inclined my ear to God's sayings. And it will work for you, too, if you will put God's Word first above every situation and circumstance that comes your way.

If you're struggling today with the tests and trials of life, stop your struggling and start inclining! Put God's Word first, and you will live the abundant life!

Questions for Study

1. God's words are full of _____, _____, and _____?

2. In Proverbs 4:20, what does the phrase ". . . attend to my WORDS . . ." mean?
   _____
   _____

3. We take God's medicine by doing four things listed in Proverbs 4:20,21. What are they?
   _____
   _____

4. In order for God's Word to do you any good, what must you do?
   _____
   _____

5. When you feed your spirit on God's Word along the lines of healing, what are you doing to your body?
   _____
   _____

6. How can we know the will of God in the situations and circumstances of life?
   _____
   _____

7. You can spare yourself a lot of misery in life by doing what?
   _____
   _____

8. What happens when you obey one part of the Bible?
   _____
   _____

9. Who is the thief that steals, kills, and destroys?
   _____
   _____

10. People who don't believe it is God's will to heal have a distorted mental picture of the character of God. How can they remedy that?
   _____
   _____

Chapter 7

Roadblocks to Healing—Part 1

The road to divine healing is seldom an expressway. More often than not, it is strewn with roadblocks placed in our way by the devil to keep us from the blessing of health that God has provided.

These roadblocks wear subtle disguises and come from many sources. Some have their basis in tradition, others in superstition. Still others are based on misquoted and misunderstood scriptures.

But God's Word clearly reveals the tactics Satan uses to keep us off the road to healing. This two-part lesson examines the seven most common roadblocks to divine healing that the believer must understand in order to remove them from his life.

Roadblock Number One: 'God Sends Sickness Upon People'

The first roadblock to healing that people encounter is the idea or teaching that God sends sickness upon people.

Some people have said that the Old Testament declares that God sent sickness upon people. Those who say this usually quote Exodus 15:26.

EXODUS 15:26
26 . . . If thou wilt diligently hearken to the voice of the Lord thy God, and wilt do that which is right in his sight, and wilt give ear to his commandments, and keep all his statutes, I will put none of these diseases upon thee, which I have brought upon the Egyptians: for I am the Lord that healeth thee.

Similar scriptures are Isaiah 45:7: *"I form the light, and create darkness: I make peace, and create evil: I the Lord do all these things,"* and Micah 1:12, which says, *"For the inhabitant of Maroth waited carefully for good: but evil came down from the Lord unto the gate of Jerusalem."*

Obviously, these passages in the *King James Version* of the Bible do not give the true meaning of the original Hebrew, for we know that God doesn't create evil. Evil can't come from Heaven, because there is no evil there. God only *permits* evil. He doesn't *create* it. Nor does He create sickness—He only permits it to come as a result of man's disobedience.

Does God Have a Purpose in Permitting Sickness?

As I've already said in previous chapters, I was healed of a deformed heart, paralysis, and an incurable blood disease as a teenager. Some folks said to me "Well, maybe God didn't exactly send the sicknesses on you, but he permitted it," implying that since He permitted it, He had some purpose in it. But just because God permits something doesn't mean He has a purpose in it.

God only permits sickness to come. Sickness is not His will. God's will is for you to walk in His statutes and keep His commandments. Then He will take sickness away from the midst of you. As I said before, sickness comes as a result of man's disobedience.

The key to understanding these different passages of Scripture lies in knowing that the active verbs in the Hebrew have been translated in the *causative* sense when they should have been translated in the *permissive* sense.

Dr. Robert Young, the author of *Young's Analytical Concordance to the Bible* and an outstanding Hebrew scholar, points this out in his book *Hints and Helps to Bible Interpretation*. He says that in Exodus 15:26, the literal Hebrew reads: ". . . I will permit to be put upon thee none of these diseases which I permitted to be brought upon the Egyptians, for I am the Lord that healeth thee."

We must bear in mind that the Bible is progressive revelation. We don't get the full revelation of the Bible in either the Old Testament or the New Testament. Neither is fully understood without the other. It's been said that "The New is in the Old concealed and the Old is in the New revealed."

So when we examine both the Old and New Testaments, we come into a full revelation of the Bible.

Where Does Sickness Come From?

We've looked at some verses of Scripture on sickness and healing in the Old Testament, now let's look at some verses in the New Testament.

First, let's take another look at Acts 10:38 and review a few things we learned in previous chapters.

ACTS 10:38
38 How God anointed Jesus of Nazareth with the Holy Ghost and with power: who went about DOING GOOD, and HEALING all that were oppressed of the devil; for God was with him.

Notice that Jesus went about doing good and healing. This important scripture shows that Jesus is the Healer and that Satan is the oppressor. This verse also points out that every person whom Jesus healed had been oppressed by the devil. As we have seen, healing is connected with doing good. Healing is a good gift from God, and healing belongs to God's children.

The Bible says, *". . . in the mouth of two or three witnesses every word may be established"* (Matt. 18:16). Let's read another account of how Jesus did good by healing one of God's children.

LUKE 13:10-17
10 And he [Jesus] was teaching in one of the synagogues on the sabbath.
11 And, behold, there was a woman which had a spirit of infirmity eighteen years, and was bowed together, and could in no wise lift up herself.
12 And when Jesus saw her, he called her to him, and said unto her, Woman, thou art loosed from thine infirmity.
13 And he laid his hands on her: and immediately she was made straight, and glorified God.
14 And the ruler of the synagogue answered with indignation, because that Jesus had healed on the sabbath day, and said unto the people, There are six days in which men ought to work: in them therefore come and be healed, and not on the sabbath day.
15 The Lord then answered him, and said, Thou hypocrite, doth not each one of you on the sabbath loose his ox or his ass from the stall, and lead him away to watering?
16 And ought not THIS WOMAN, being a daughter of Abraham, WHOM SATAN HATH BOUND, lo, these eighteen years, be loosed from this bond on the sabbath day?
17 And when he had said these things, all his adversaries were ashamed: and all the people rejoiced for all the glorious things that were done by him.

Verse 16 plainly tells us that *Satan* was the one who bound the woman with sickness for all those years. But *Jesus* was the One who healed her!

Then First John 3:8 tells us that Jesus was manifested to destroy the works of the devil. And the New Testament makes it clear that *sickness* is a work of the devil.

Here's further proof that sickness is the work of the devil:

JOHN 10:10
10 The thief [Satan] cometh not, but for to steal, and to kill, and to destroy: I [Jesus] am come that they might have life, and that they might have it more abundantly.

Jesus didn't come to destroy. He's not the destroyer; Satan is! You need to understand that fact, because if you think that God will put sickness on you for some divine or supernatural purpose, then that roadblock will stand between you and your healing.

Remember that when God commanded Moses to go down into Egypt and lead the children of Israel out of bondage, He sent Moses to plead with Pharaoh to release the people. God didn't *want* the plagues to come upon the Egyptian people. But when Pharaoh hardened his heart, God withdrew His protecting hand and permitted the plagues to sweep over the land of Egypt.

When the final plague—death, the messenger of hell—was permitted, death went forth and destroyed the firstborn of every Egyptian household. Only then was Pharaoh compelled to yield and let the children of Israel go.

Where did the plague of death come from? Did it come from Heaven? Are there any dead in Heaven? The answer to these questions is no, of course. Death has never entered there, and it will never enter there. There will be no death in Heaven (Rev. 21:4)!

God is not the author of death; He's the author of life. God hates death. Where does death come from, then? It comes from Satan, who has the power of death.

HEBREWS 2:14
14 Forasmuch then as the children are partakers of flesh and blood, he [Jesus] also himself likewise took part of the same; that through death he might destroy him that had the power of death, that is, the devil.

You see, the law of sin and death is the *devil's* law. But the law of the Spirit of life in Christ Jesus is *God's* law. Romans 8:2 says, *"For the law of the Spirit of life in Christ Jesus hath made me free from the law of sin and death."* Death is our final enemy. And we have the promise that when Jesus comes again, this last enemy shall be put underfoot (1 Cor. 15:26).

Christ came to destroy "him that had the power of death" (Heb. 2:14). Satan isn't destroyed yet, but he will be put in the bottomless pit for a thousand years after Jesus returns. After the end of all things, Satan will be put in the lake of fire and brimstone forever (Rev. 20:10)!

So the plague of death that came upon Egypt did not come until God withdrew His hand of protection and permitted it. His permission, however, should not be confused with commission. For example, God *permits* people to establish bars and nightclubs. He *permits* people to steal and kill. But He certainly doesn't *commission* those actions. There is a vast difference between *permission* and *commission*.

Now on the Day of Pentecost, Peter declared that Christ was crucified by the hands of wicked men: *"Him [Jesus] . . . ye have taken, and by wicked hands have crucified and slain"* (Acts 2:23). In other words, it was the devil's work done by his own children.

When the Pharisees stirred up the high priesthood against Jesus, He said, *"Ye are of your father the devil, and the lusts of your father ye will do . . ."* (John 8:44). It was not the work

of God that the Pharisees turned people against Jesus, even though God permitted it.

But the fact that God permits wickedness doesn't mean that people have to commit sinful acts, any more than it means that people have to turn against Christ. Many people are crucifying Jesus afresh today because they are rejecting Him. Yet God doesn't commission them to reject Him; He just permits them to make their own choice—He gave man the free will to accept or reject His Son.

Roadblock Number Two: 'My Healing May Not Be God's Will'

The second roadblock to healing that people encounter is: "My healing may not be God's will."

When some people pray for healing, they think they should pray, "If it be Thy will." Many times that's the reason their prayers don't work—they're using the wrong method of prayer.

There was only one instance when Jesus ever prayed that way. When Jesus was in the Garden of Gethsemane, He prayed a *prayer of consecration* and *dedication*. That's not the same as a *prayer of petition* or asking God for something.

In Matthew 26:39, when Jesus *". . . fell on his face, and prayed, saying, O my Father, if it be possible, let this cup pass from me: nevertheless not as I will, but as thou wilt,"* He was dedicating Himself to the will of God. Jesus prayed this prayer the same way we might pray, "Lord, I'll go wherever You want me to go. If You want me to go to Africa, I'll go."

But when the Bible already tells us God's will for us, we don't have to pray, "If it be Thy will." For example, if a man's rent is due and his children need food to eat, he doesn't have to pray, "Lord, if it's Your will, please supply my needs." Why? Because the Bible says, *". . . my God shall supply all your need according to his riches in glory by Christ Jesus"* (Phil. 4:19)! That man should pray and believe God to meet his needs.

Some people just tack the phrase "If it be Thy will" on the end of their prayers out of tradition. They think they're being humble, but they're really robbing themselves of the blessings of God. Anything the Bible promises you or says belongs to you is yours. You don't have to put an "if" in your prayers when you pray according to God's Word!

That's why praying, "Lord, if it be Thy will, please heal me" is unnecessary. God has plainly told us in His Word that it *is* His will to heal us.

A sinner wouldn't pray, "Lord, save me, *if it be Thy will*." That kind of prayer would be ridiculous, because God's Word declares that He is *". . . not willing that any should perish, but that all should come to repentance"* (2 Peter 3:9). God's Word also states that *". . . whosoever will, let him take the water of life freely"* (Rev. 22:17). Therefore, the sinner doesn't have to pray *"If it be Thy will."*

Similarly, it is just as ridiculous for a child of God to pray, "Lord, *heal* me, if it be Thy will." Why? Because the Bible tells us that Jesus already paid the price for our healing!

MATTHEW 8:17
17 That it might be fulfilled which was spoken by Esaias the prophet, saying, Himself [Jesus] **took our infirmities, and bare our sicknesses.**

Now just because you read Matthew 8:17 doesn't mean it's going to work for you. A lot of times people think the Word is just going to work for them automatically. For example, some Christians who know that the Bible says Jesus *". . . took our infirmities, and bare our sicknesses"* (Matt. 8:17), expect the results of that verse to just fall on them. They say, "Well, if that verse is so, why don't I have divine health?" They're not experiencing divine healing and health because they don't really believe and accept God's Word. The truth of God's Word won't do them any good until they *know* it, *believe* it, and *accept* it.

It's hard for some people to see what the Scriptures are really saying because they've been "religiously trained" instead of scripturally taught. In other words, they read the Bible with glasses colored with religious tradition.

I know, because I had to read Matthew 8:17 over and over again myself before I thoroughly understood it. But when I fully understood what this verse really meant, I rejoiced in it, for then I was able to emphasize the word "our." He took *our* infirmities and bore *our* sicknesses—and I am included in that word "our." Therefore, I can say that He took *my* infirmities and bore *my* sicknesses.

That brings it right down to where I live! In other words, I don't have to bear my sicknesses anymore, because *Jesus* bore them that I might be free!

When I made this discovery, I decided there wasn't any need for both Jesus *and* me to bear my sicknesses. And if Jesus bore them that I might be free, why should I pray, "if it be Thy will"? The Bible states that it *is* His will!

Most people who don't believe in divine healing stay away from Matthew 8:17. However, occasionally a brave soul will come up with what he thinks is the answer to this scripture once and for all.

One person said this verse meant that Christ took the sicknesses of the people who lived at that time, but it doesn't apply to us today. But he forgot that Matthew wrote his Gospel *after* Jesus died. If healing had applied only to those living while Jesus was on this earth in the flesh, Matthew would have written, "He Himself took *their* infirmities and bare *their* sicknesses." However, Matthew didn't write it that way. The Holy Spirit, through Matthew, wrote, "He Himself took *our* infirmities and bare *our* sicknesses."

Someone else advanced the theory that this particular verse doesn't refer to the past, but refers to the future; therefore, it will come to pass during the Millennium. That can't be true, however, because there will be no need for healing then. Why? Because the curse will be lifted!

Paul said we will all be changed, *"In a moment, in the twinkling of an eye . . ."* (1 Cor. 15:52). We'll have new bodies fashioned like unto Jesus' glorious body (Phil. 3:21). Our bodies won't be plagued with sickness during the Millennium, so we will not need this provision for healing then.

No, the promise of divine healing belongs to us *now*—because we are subject to sickness in this life, not in the life that is to come. The promise that Jesus Christ took our infirmities and bore our sicknesses belongs to us today. Therefore, we don't need to pray, "If it be Thy will." God's Word has clearly shown us His will.

Still, someone else might ask, without quoting the entire verse, "But didn't Christ teach us to pray in Matthew 6:10, 'Father, Thy will be done'?" However, to use just one portion of that scripture is to use only half a truth. And as someone else said, "Beware of the half-truth. You may have gotten the wrong half!"

Christ taught us to pray, "Thy will be done in earth *as it is in Heaven*." As I said in a previous chapter, Jesus wasn't teaching us to pray, "If it be Thy will" when it comes to healing. He was teaching us to pray that God's will might be done here on earth just as it is done in Heaven. There is no sickness or disease in Heaven. So if it's not His will that there be sickness and disease in Heaven, then it's not His will that there be sickness and disease on earth. If His will is truly done on earth as it is done in Heaven, there will be no sickness or disease among us.

Again, when it comes to divine healing, people have all kinds of different ideas. Some people don't believe in divine healing at all. While others say, "God can heal, if it's His will. And it might be His will to heal some people or some sicknesses, but not all of them."

A man once told me he knew it wasn't God's will to heal a certain condition in his body because of an experience he had. He explained saying, just as he awoke one morning, his room lit up and someone in a long white robe appeared to him. He thought it was Jesus, although he did not see the person's face. The person said to him, "It is not my will to heal you," and then he disappeared. Ever since then, the man had accepted the idea that it wasn't God's will to heal him.

I asked him, "What if one of your unsaved loved ones told you that through a similar incident, God had revealed to him that it was not His will to save him? You would immediately point out scriptures to prove to him that it's not God's will for anyone to perish, but that all should come to repentance (2 Peter 3:9; John 3:16). You would explain that the person he mistook for Jesus was really a messenger of Satan, for Jesus wouldn't contradict His own Word, would He?"

I got that man to see that Jesus had already taken his infirmities and borne his sicknesses, and he got healed! Praise God!

Satan will try to defeat us every way he can. That's why it's so important that we know what the Word says. I tell you, we can be just as certain that divine healing is God's will as we are that saving the lost is His will. And we know it by knowing His Word. God's Word is His will.

The same Bible that gives us John 3:16 also says, *"Surely he hath borne our griefs* [sicknesses]*, and carried our sorrows* [diseases]*: yet we did esteem him stricken, smitten of God, and afflicted. But he was wounded for OUR transgressions, he was bruised for OUR iniquities: the chastisement of OUR peace was upon him; and with his stripes WE ARE HEALED"* (Isa. 53:4,5).

Remember, the Old Testament was originally written in Hebrew. And the Hebrew words for the words translated "griefs" and "sorrows" in the *King James Version* of this verse mean *sicknesses* and *diseases*.

The Bible also says that Jesus *". . . bare our sins in his own body on the tree, that we, being dead to sins, should live unto righteousness: by whose stripes ye were healed"* (1 Peter 2:24).

That's good news! Jesus Christ is the same yesterday, today, and forever (Heb. 13:8). He never changes. He can and *will* make believers whole today!

We're discussing the seven most common roadblocks to healing. We've seen that sickness and disease do not come from God, and that God doesn't use sickness and disease to teach people a lesson. We've also seen that it is God's will to heal *every* illness and infirmity. We'll continue our discussion of these roadblocks in the next chapter.

Questions for Study

1. What is the basis of the roadblocks the devil uses to keep us from enjoying the blessing of health that God has provided?

   _____

   _____

2. Name the two roadblocks discussed in this chapter.

   _____

   _____

3. Some people say that Exodus 15:26, Isaiah 45:7, and Micah 1:12 declare that God sent sickness upon people. Why is it obvious that these passages in the King James Version of the Bible don't give the true meaning of the original Hebrew?

   _____

   _____

4. Why does God permit sickness?

   _____

   _____

5. What was the final plague that God permitted to sweep over the land of Egypt?

   _____

   _____

6. Complete this sentence: God is the author of _____.

7. What is our final enemy?

   _____

   _____

8. When some people pray for healing, they think they should pray, "If it be Thy will." Why is that prayer unnecessary?

   _____

   _____

9. When did Matthew write his Gospel?

   _____

   _____

10. Why does the promise of divine healing belong to us now?

    _____

    _____

Chapter 8

Roadblocks to Healing—Part 2

The previous chapter covered two of the most common roadblocks to healing. In this chapter we will deal with five more roadblocks the devil uses to try to keep people from enjoying their God-given right to divine healing and health.

Roadblock Number Three: 'Hezekiah Used a Poultice'

The third roadblock to healing that people encounter is: "Hezekiah used a poultice."

ISAIAH 38:1-5
1   In those days was Hezekiah sick unto death. And Isaiah the prophet the son of Amoz came unto him, and said unto him, Thus saith the Lord, Set thine house in order: for thou shalt die, and not live.
2   Then Hezekiah turned his face toward the wall, and prayed unto the Lord,
3   And said, Remember now, O Lord, I beseech thee, how I have walked before thee in truth and with a perfect heart, and have done that which is good in thy sight. And Hezekiah wept sore.
4   Then came the word of the Lord to Isaiah, saying,
5   Go, and say to Hezekiah, Thus saith the Lord, the God of David thy father, I have heard thy prayer, I have seen thy tears: behold, I will add unto thy days fifteen years.

We read later in verses 20 and 21 that Hezekiah said: *"The Lord was ready to save me: therefore we will sing my songs to the stringed instruments all the days of our life in the house of the Lord. For Isaiah had said, Let them take a lump of figs, and lay it for a plaister upon the boil, and he shall recover."*

Some have wondered why God told Hezekiah to put a lump or poultice of figs on the boil. One very able Bible scholar who was a medical doctor, minister, and Hebrew student says that according to the Hebrew translation, Hezekiah had a carbuncle on his neck, which can be very serious.

God already told Hezekiah that he would not die but would live for fifteen more years. Therefore, the poultice of figs was not necessary as a medicinal aid. It had no curative powers whatsoever. It served no medical purpose.

Sometimes It Takes an Act of Obedience To Release Your Faith

Many people through the years have used different poultices as cleansing agents, and some feel that Hezekiah's poultice may have been used in this manner. I am convinced, however, that God told Hezekiah to lay a lump of figs on the boil as an act of obedience and faith, just as He told Naaman the leper to dip in the Jordan River seven times so that his leprosy would be cleansed. Dipping in the muddy Jordan didn't have any curative value. It didn't heal Naaman any more than the poultice healed Hezekiah.

In my own ministry, the Spirit of God will lead me at times to tell sick people to do something as an act of faith. For example, in one service the Lord led me to minister to some people who were crippled. He didn't tell me to pray for them or to lay hands on them. He directed me to tell them to run.

Well, the first man who came up for healing couldn't even lift his feet off the floor. He just scooted along and stood with his knees bent. It looked as if he were still sitting down, because his knees were drawn up. When I asked him if he could run, it startled him. He answered, "Oh, my God, no. I can't even walk, much less run."

Then I told him that the Lord had shown me that if he would run, he would be healed. I never saw anyone turn around and scoot away so fast in my life! That fellow took off and scooted down one aisle and back up the other as fast as he could go. When he returned to the platform, he was still scooting. He wasn't a bit better.

I told him to do it again, and this time I went with him—up one aisle and down the other. When he got back this time he was perfectly healed and walking as normally as I was! God had told him to do something seemingly impossible as an act of faith and obedience, and the Lord honored his simple faith.

When the Spirit of God tells someone to do a certain thing, it usually involves an act of obedience to release that person's faith. That doesn't mean that everyone who does what the Lord tells a certain person to do will be healed. But it does mean that if God says for you to do something and you act upon it, you will be healed.

Roadblock Number Four: 'Paul Left Trophimus Sick at Miletum'

The fourth roadblock to healing that people encounter is: "Paul left Trophimus sick at Miletum."

2 TIMOTHY 4:20
20 Erastus abode at Corinth: but Trophimus have I [Paul] left at Miletum sick.

Some quoting this verse argue that divine healing must not always be God's will since Paul left Trophimus sick at Miletum. But they fail to understand that Paul did not carry healing power around with him. Trophimus' faith played a part in his healing.

Your Faith Plays a Role in Your Receiving Healing

Healing is primarily a faith proposition on the part of the individual who receives. No matter how much faith a minister may have, the effects of an individual's doubt will nullify that minister's faith.

This is another area where some folks have made a great mistake. They think that if a minister has faith and he prays the prayer of faith for them, they'll get healed—whether *they* have faith or not.

Even under Jesus' ministry not everyone was healed. On one occasion in his own hometown of Nazareth, only a few people received healing.

MARK 6:1-6
1 And he [Jesus] went out from thence, and came into his own country; and his disciples follow him.

2 And when the sabbath day was come, he began to teach in the synagogue: and many hearing him were astonished, saying, From whence hath this man these things? and what wisdom is this which is given unto him, that even such mighty works are wrought by his hands?
3 Is not this the carpenter, the son of Mary, the brother of James, and Joses, and of Juda, and Simon? and are not his sisters here with us? And they were offended at him.
4 But Jesus said unto them, A prophet is not without honour, but in his own country, and among his own kin, and in his own house.
5 And he could there do no mighty work, save that he laid his hands upon a few sick folk, and healed them.
6 And he marvelled because of their unbelief. And he went round about the villages, teaching.

The original Greek translation of verse 5 says that Jesus laid hands on a few sick folk with minor ailments and healed them. So in this case, the few who did get healed only had minor things wrong with them. Well, why couldn't Jesus heal everyone there who needed healing? Because of their unbelief (v. 6)!

You see, Jesus couldn't just override their unbelief. Someone might ask, "But isn't Jesus the Son of God? Isn't He Sovereign?" Emphatically, yes! But Jesus can't override someone's unbelief. He won't do it. He would have to violate His Word to do that. So how did Jesus help people? He went around their villages teaching them the Word of God to cure their unbelief.

In nearly every one of my meetings, there are some people who don't receive their healing. But many people do get healed. Just because some do not, doesn't mean that it's not God's will that they be healed.

That's the reason I said that healing is primarily a faith proposition on the part of the individual who receives.

The Bible says, *"Can two walk together, except they be agreed?"* (Amos 3:3). And Jesus said in Matthew 18:19, *". . . if two of you shall agree on earth as touching any thing that they shall ask, it shall be done for them of my Father which is in heaven."* (The negative side of this verse would be, of course, that if they don't agree, it won't be done.) Your faith plays a part in your healing.

Healings vs. Miracles

In his writings, Paul differentiated between miracles and healing. Miracles involving healing are instantaneous healings. Other healings are gradual, but they are still of God. For example, the Bible says that when Jesus prayed for the nobleman's son, the boy began to amend from that hour (John 4:46-53). It may be that when Paul left Trophimus, Trophimus was still sick from all outward appearances, but the healing process had already begun.

In 1953, a 28-year-old man who had never walked in his life was brought to a service I was holding in Dallas, Texas. Doctors who had examined him could find no physical reason for his inability to walk. As far as they could tell, he was normal.

As I laid hands on him, the Lord showed me that an evil spirit oppressed his body. This was the reason doctors could not help him. I rebuked that spirit. Then I told the young man that the demon that had been oppressing him was gone and that he could walk.

I knew he would not get up and start walking immediately; his healing would come gradually. A year and a half later, I was back in Dallas and learned that the young man was walking everywhere on his own.

Often gradual healings are greater than instant healings, because some people who are quickly healed forget God. On the other hand, those who are healed gradually as they continue to believe God's Word often develop strong faith.

Roadblock Number Five: 'Paul Had a Thorn in the Flesh'

The fifth roadblock to healing that people encounter is: "Paul had a thorn in the flesh."

2 CORINTHIANS 12:7-10

7   And lest I [Paul] should be exalted above measure through the abundance of the revelations, there was given to me a thorn in the flesh, the messenger of Satan to buffet me, lest I should be exalted above measure.

8   For this thing I besought the Lord thrice, that it might depart from me.

9   And he said unto me, My grace is sufficient for thee: for my strength is made perfect in weakness. Most gladly therefore will I rather glory in my infirmities, that the power of Christ may rest upon me.

10 Therefore I take pleasure in infirmities, in reproaches, in necessities, in persecutions, in distresses for Christ's sake: for when I am weak, then am I strong.

Because of this passage of Scripture, the thought is widely held that Paul had a sickness which God refused to heal. This teaching has led many to believe that it must be God's will for some of His saints to be sick, and it has held people in bondage when they should be delivered.

One common belief is that Paul suffered from some disease of the eyes and was nearly blind. The Bible states that the Lord Jesus appeared to Ananias in a vision and told him to go lay hands on Saul (Paul) that he might receive his sight. Ananias did and God healed Saul (Acts 9:12-18). Therefore, to conclude that Paul had eye trouble because of that brief blindness would be to belittle the work of God.

Also, when Paul was on the island of Melita, he preached to the people and told them about the redemptive work of God. If his eyes had been full of pus, as some claim, would those people have believed God for healing? Yet the Bible says that when Paul laid hands on them, they were healed (Acts 28:8,9).

What Was Paul's Thorn in the Flesh?

It is true that God permitted this "thorn in the flesh" to come upon Paul, but it was not from God. The scripture says that a "messenger of Satan was permitted to buffet him." *The Bible does not say that this thorn in the flesh was a sickness.*

I mentioned in a previous chapter that the expression "thorn in the flesh" is used elsewhere in the Bible. Before the children of Israel went into Canaan's land, God told them to destroy the inhabitants of the country, the Canaanites. He said if they didn't destroy the Canaanites, it would cause them trouble in the future—the Canaanites would be a thorn in their side.

NUMBERS 33:55
55 But if ye will not drive out the inhabitants of the land from before you; then it shall come to pass, that those which ye let remain of them shall be pricks in your eyes, and thorns in your sides, and shall vex you in the land wherein ye dwell.

There is no reference to sickness in this scripture at all. Neither was Paul's thorn sickness. It was a messenger of Satan to buffet him. Everywhere Paul went, the devil stirred up strife against him.

Paul wrote of the many times he had been whipped and imprisoned. He was even stoned and left for dead. Yet in all of his writings about persecutions and tribulations, not once does he include sickness among them. Nowhere in the Scriptures do we find where Paul was ever disabled by sickness during his ministry.

What Purpose Did Paul's Thorn Serve?

Why, then, did God permit this thorn in the flesh to buffet Paul? The Scriptures say it was to keep Paul from developing a tendency to be prideful about the revelations and visions he'd had (2 Cor. 12:7).

Before anyone claims that he has a "thorn in the flesh," it might be well to ask how many revelations and visions he has had! Most people who think they have a thorn in the flesh haven't had any kind of revelation or vision. They're simply permitting Satan to defeat them and keep them from the blessings of God because of their ignorance and doubt.

However, there are some who do have a thorn in the flesh in some of the ways Paul did, because the devil is ever present to stir up trouble and hinder them in the work they are doing for God. But notice that God said, ". . . *My grace is sufficient for thee . . .*" (2 Cor. 12:9). Glory to God! *God's grace gives us power to rise above the buffetings of Satan.*

Roadblock Number Six: 'I'm Suffering for the Glory of God'

The sixth roadblock to healing that people encounter is: "I'm suffering for the glory of God."

Those who support this belief usually point to the scripture in John chapter 9, when Jesus passed by a man who had been born blind.

JOHN 9:1-4
1 And as Jesus passed by, he saw a man which was blind from his birth.
2 And his disciples asked him, saying, Master, who did sin, this man, or his parents, that he was born blind?
3 Jesus answered, Neither hath this man sinned, nor his parents: but that the works of God should be made manifest in him.
4 I must work the works of him that sent me, while it is day: the night cometh, when no man can work.

Jesus' disciples asked Him who had sinned and caused the man to be blind—the man or his parents? Jesus said, ". . . *Neither hath this man sinned, nor his parents: but that THE WORKS OF GOD should be made manifest in him*" (v. 3).

Therefore, some people reason from this verse that the man was born blind in order that God might get glory from it. But Jesus went on to say, "*I must work the works of him that sent me, while it is day: the night cometh, when no man can work*" (v. 4).

Well, the works of God weren't made manifest in that blind man until Christ did what He was sent to do. Jesus healed the man's blindness. So "the works" that Jesus was referring to was *healing*, not the man's blindness.

What About Lazarus?

Someone might ask, "What about Lazarus? Doesn't the Bible say he was sick for the glory of God?" No, people just put their own interpretation on that. Remember when Jesus got word that Lazarus was sick? Jesus purposely tarried instead of hurrying to His friend's bedside. Then He told His disciples: ". . . *This sickness is not unto death, but for the glory of God, that the Son of God might be glorified thereby*" (John 11: 4).

Later when Jesus arrived in Bethany with His disciples, Lazarus had been dead four days. Lazarus' sister Martha told Jesus that if He had been there, her brother would not have died. Then Jesus told her that her brother would rise again.

JOHN 11:24-26

24 Martha saith unto him [Jesus], I know that he [Lazarus] shall rise again in the resurrection at the last day.

25 Jesus said unto her, I am the resurrection, and the life: he that believeth in me, though he were dead, yet shall he live:

26 And whosoever liveth and believeth in me shall never die. Believest thou this?

Shortly after this, Martha protested Christ's command to roll away Lazarus' gravestone. She knew that after four days, Lazarus' body would have already begun to decompose and stink. But notice Jesus' response: "*. . . Said I not unto thee, that, if thou wouldest believe, thou shouldest see THE GLORY OF GOD?*" (v. 40).

Jesus was really telling Martha that she had not yet seen the glory of God. Martha couldn't have seen the glory of God in her brother's death, because God's glory hadn't been made manifest yet. The glory of God was not manifested in Lazarus' being sick and dying. The glory of God was manifested in Lazarus' resurrection and healing! (Lazarus not only had to be *resurrected*, but he also had to be *healed* of whatever had caused his death. If he wasn't also healed, he would have died again immediately.)

God is glorified through healing and deliverance, not through sickness and suffering!

Roadblock Number Seven: 'Sickness Is God's Chastening'

The seventh roadblock to healing that people encounter is: "Sickness is God's chastening."

It is true that the Bible says, *"For whom the Lord loveth he chasteneth . . ."* (Heb. 12:6). However, it does not say, "Whom the Lord loveth He maketh sick!"

It is a mistake to take a small portion of Scripture and try to prove something. There is no reference to sickness in this text, and there is no implication of sickness or disease in the word "chasteneth" in the original Greek.

As we studied previously, the full meaning of this word can be gleaned from the writings of Dr. Robert Young, a recognized Greek scholar, and

W. E. Vine, author of *An Expository Dictionary of New Testament Words.*

We learn from them that "chasten" literally means *to child train*, *educate*, or *teach*. Just as babies need to be taught and corrected so that they can grow to be healthy children and adults, baby Christians need to be taught and corrected so that they can grow to be spiritually healthy Christians. God's children need to be disciplined and governed, which is what the word "chasten" means in the original Greek.

How Does God Chasten His Children?

Children must be disciplined, corrected, and trained in love. As we said, one meaning of the word "chasten" is *to educate*. Parents send their children to school so they can be educated. But, again, parents don't tell the teacher, "If my child doesn't act right, just knock his eye out or break his leg." That isn't the way to educate a child. And that's not how God educates His children either!

MATTHEW 7:7-11

7 Ask, and it shall be given you; seek, and ye shall find; knock, and it shall be opened unto you:

8 For every one that asketh receiveth; and he that seeketh findeth; and to him that knocketh it shall be opened.

9 Or what man is there of you, whom if his son ask bread, will he give him a stone?

10 Or if he ask a fish, will he give him a serpent?

11 If ye then, being evil, know how to give good gifts unto your children, how much more shall your Father which is in heaven give good things to them that ask him?

You wouldn't need any other scripture in the Bible to preach divine healing (and we have plenty of them) than verse 11. Let me show you what I mean. How many of you parents want your children to be sick? Not one of you. You'll do everything in the world that you can to provide for them so that your children will eat well, live well, and stay well.

Well, what is Jesus saying in Matthew 7:7-11? He's saying that if earthly parents, who are carnal, know how to give good gifts to their children, how much more will our Heavenly Father give *good* things! God gives His children beyond what earthly parents could even think or do! That's because *"Every good gift and every perfect gift is from above, and cometh down from the Father of lights, with whom is no variableness, neither shadow of turning"* (James 1:17). God doesn't change. He always gives good gifts!

We've already learned that healing is connected with doing good. The Bible says, *"How God anointed Jesus of Nazareth with the Holy Ghost and with power: who went about DOING GOOD, AND HEALING all that were oppressed of the devil; for God was with him"* (Acts 10:38).

The Bible tells us that healing is good, but we don't have to read the Bible to know that's true. We just have good sense, we know that.

Have you ever been sick? Have you ever been well? Which one is better? Being well is much better, isn't it? Healing is a good gift from God, and healing belongs to God's children!

Questions for Study

1. Name the five roadblocks to healing discussed in this chapter.

   _____

   _____

2. How many years did God say He would add to King Hezekiah's life?

   _____

   _____

3. When the Spirit of God tells someone to do a certain thing, what is usually involved in releasing that person's faith?

   _____

   _____

4. Healing is primarily a faith proposition on the part of whom?

   _____

   _____

5. What is the difference between miracles and healing?

   _____

   _____

6. According to Second Corinthians 12:7, what was Paul's thorn in the flesh?

   _____

   _____

7. Why did God permit this thorn in the flesh to buffet Paul?

   _____

   _____

8. What are the "works of God" that Jesus referred to in John 9:3?

   _____

   _____

9. What is the literal meaning of the word "chasten"?

   _____

   _____

10. What do baby Christians need to grow to be spiritually healthy Christians?

    _____

    _____

Chapter 9

Spiritual Healing?

In God's plan of redemption, not only is there the remission of sin, Jesus also provided healing for our physical bodies. The Bible contains many scriptures that prove Jesus not only carried our sins on the cross, but our sicknesses as well.

MATTHEW 8:17
17 That it might be fulfilled which was spoken by Esaias the prophet, saying, Himself took our infirmities, and bare our sicknesses.

ISAIAH 53:4
4 Surely he hath borne our griefs, and carried our sorrows: yet we did esteem him stricken, smitten of God, and afflicted.

1 PETER 2:24
24 Who his own self bare our sins in his own body on the tree, that we, being dead to sins, should live unto righteousness: by whose stripes ye were healed.

In our first text, Matthew is quoting Isaiah, saying, *". . . Himself took our infirmities, and bare our sicknesses."* Let's take a closer look at the passage Matthew quotes from Isaiah.

I call Isaiah chapter 53 "The great redemptive chapter." In this chapter, we see Isaiah prophesying about the coming Messiah, the Lord Jesus Christ. Isaiah 53:4 is a verse that should be familiar to you since we've studied it in previous chapters.

ISAIAH 53:4
4 Surely he [Jesus] hath borne our griefs, and carried our sorrows: yet we did esteem him stricken, smitten of God, and afflicted.

Isaiah 53:4 says, *"Surely he hath borne our GRIEFS, and carried our SORROWS. . . ."* Again, this translation is from the *King James Version*. But as the marginal notes in many study Bibles point out, a more accurate translation of the words "griefs" and "sorrows" would have been "diseases" and "pains." So in the original Hebrew, this verse actually reads: "Surely He—Jesus—hath borne our *diseases* and carried our *pains*. . . ."

This is the way Dr. Isaac Leeser translated those two Hebrew words for his Orthodox Jewish translation of the Bible. But you really don't need to know anything about Hebrew in order to gain a clear understanding of what this scripture meant, because you can simply read what Matthew said about Jesus, quoting Isaiah: *". . . Himself took our INFIRMITIES, and bare our SICKNESSES"* (Matt. 8:17).

Let's go back to Isaiah chapter 53 for a moment. Verse 10 reads: *"Yet it pleased the Lord to bruise him; he hath put him to grief. . . ."* Where the *King James Version* says, *". . . he hath put him to grief . . ."* other translations say, "he hath made him sick." According to this verse, God delighted to bruise Jesus and make Him sick. Why? Because it meant healing for all mankind!

Jesus Christ bore our sins and paid the penalty that we might be free from sin. He also bore our diseases and carried our pains that we wouldn't have to bear them.

After I read in my Bible that Jesus Himself took my infirmities and bare my sicknesses, I decided there wasn't any need for both Him and me to bear them, and I've been free from sickness ever since!

In our third text, First Peter 2:24, we read, *"Who his own self [Jesus] bare our sins in his own body on the tree, that we, being dead to sins, should live unto righteousness: BY WHOSE STRIPES YE WERE HEALED."* Here Peter is looking back to the sacrifice of Christ when he says, "by whose stripes ye were healed." Notice that "were healed" is past tense.

Now consider those last two scriptures together: "Himself took our infirmities and bare our sicknesses; by whose stripes you were healed."

That verse in First Peter has been misunderstood by many in the past, so I want to look at it closely for a moment. I was reading after a supposedly outstanding Bible scholar who said,

"First Peter 2:24 doesn't mean physical healing; it's referring to spiritual healing: 'By whose stripes you were healed *spiritually.'*"

Now this man was supposed to be a great authority on the Scriptures. But he must not have been reading the same Bible that I was reading. According to Second Corinthians 5:17, a sinner does not get healed spiritually.

2 CORINTHIANS 5:17
17 Therefore if any man be in Christ, he is a new creature: old things are passed away; behold, all things are become new.

The human spirit of the lost man or woman is not healed—it's *reborn*. Second Corinthians 5:17 says that once a person is in Christ Jesus, he becomes a *new* creature. Old things are passed away and all things become new. So First Peter 2:24 does not refer to spiritual healing.

Dispelling the 'Spiritual Healing' Myth

If you stop to think about it, there is no such thing as *spiritual healing* mentioned in the Bible. The concept of spiritual healing probably came into being when some psychologists got saved and filled with the Holy Spirit, and then they tried to consolidate the teachings of the Bible with psychology. They were born again and filled with the Spirit, all right—wonderful, sincere Christians—but they got confused.

You see, when your body gets healed, you are just healed of a sickness or disease. You don't get a brand-new body, do you? No, of course not. You still have the same body you had before you were healed. You just got healed of the sickness or disease that afflicted your body.

Well, similarly, if your spirit were healed when you got born again, you would still have the same spirit too. It would just be healed. But the Scriptures don't teach that at all.

The Bible says that if any man is in Christ, he is a new creature. Old things are passed away and all things become new—not half of them, *all* of them (2 Cor. 5:17)! This verse is clearly talking about the *inward* man not the *outward* man.

When you're born again, you're not the same spirit that you once were.

Jesus explained the New Birth to Nicodemus, a Pharisee and ruler of the Jews, saying "*. . . Except a man be born again, he cannot see the kingdom of God*" (John 3:3). Then Nicodemus, being natural, could only think naturally, so he asked Jesus, "Is it possible for a man when he is old to enter the second time into his mother's womb and be born?" Jesus answered, "*. . . Except a man be born of water and of the Spirit, he cannot enter into the kingdom of God. That which is born of the flesh is flesh; and that which is born of the Spirit is spirit*" (vv. 5,6).

In other words, there is a natural birth whereby the flesh is born; and there is a spiritual birth whereby the spirit is born. You see, when a baby is born into this natural world, we don't say he was healed. No! We say he was born. In the same way, when a person becomes a new creature in Christ, his human spirit is not healed; it is born again.

While we're on this subject, let me also say that when a person is born again, his *soul* doesn't become new either. That's another place where folks miss it: They don't distinguish between the soul and the spirit, because they think that they are the same. But the soul and the spirit are different. In fact, man has a three-fold nature. According to the Bible, man is a spirit who possesses a soul and lives in a body (1 Thess. 5:23). The soul of man is the mind, will, and emotions.

Many people have missed it because we talk about the soul being saved when a person gets born again. James 1:21 does say: "*Wherefore lay apart all filthiness and superfluity of naughtiness, and receive with meekness the engrafted word, which is able to SAVE YOUR SOULS.*" But we've taken that verse out of context. Here the word "save" means *to renew* or *to restore*. Psalm 23:3 says that God restores your soul and Romans 12:2 says that you must renew your mind with the Word of God. Your soul can't be born again. The spirit is *reborn*, but the soul is *renewed* or *restored*.

Notice what Ezekiel prophesied under the Old Covenant:

EZEKIEL 36:26
26 A new heart also will I give you, and a new spirit will I put within you: and I will take away the stony heart out of your flesh, and I will give you an heart of flesh.

In this verse, God was saying, "The time is coming when I'll establish the New Covenant, and I'll take out that old stony heart and put a new spirit within you. Then I'm going to put My Spirit in you."

Healing Is Part of God's Redemptive Plan

That's why when I read where that fellow had said the Bible was referring to spiritual healing, I thought to myself, *Well, if that's the case, God made a mistake down there in Oklahoma!*

I mentioned in a previous chapter that during a meeting I held in Oklahoma years ago, a little 72-year-old woman was healed. The best doctors in the state said she would never walk another step the longest day she lived. She had been confined to a wheelchair for four long years.

When she was brought to my meeting, I just laid my Bible on her lap and had her read First Peter 2:24. And in ten minutes' time, she was jumping around, healed!

So if that verse meant spiritual healing, then God made a mistake. He ought to have healed her spiritually. But He healed her physically.

No, bless God, First Peter 2:24 means just what it says: "By whose stripes, ye were healed." That's talking about the healing of our human body, not our spirit!

There is only one sense in which divine healing could be called spiritual healing—if "spiritual" is being used to describe the work of God.

You see, in referring to divine healing, God is the One who heals your body, and He is a spirit (John 4:24). Therefore, in that sense you could say divine healing is spiritual healing. But that is not talking about the healing of the human spirit.

To put it another way, divine healing does not refer to being healed spiritually. However, it is spiritual because it refers to being healed *by the power of God.*

True Spiritual Healing

In ministering the tangible healing power of God, I have laid hands on people and felt the power of God go into them—then come right back out. Why? Because they didn't take hold of it!

This usually happens because folks are trying to receive healing with their mind. But divine healing is not mental. You can't contact God with your mind because He is not a mind. He is a spirit.

You see, when man heals (and man can heal, whether you realize it or not), he must either do it through the mind or through the physical senses. But when God comes on the scene as the Healer, He heals through the person's spirit.

Let me explain. God contacts us through our *spirit*, not through our mind or body—because, as we said, God is not a mind. Likewise, He is not a man (Num. 23:19). Although He has a spirit-body over in the spirit world—angels do too—God is not a *physical being*. He is a *spirit*. Therefore, He contacts us through our spirit, just as we contact Him through our spirit.

Now when God heals, He does heal *physically*, but it's through the human spirit or man's heart, where faith dwells. You see, God heals people through their faith—and the Bible says that faith is of the heart, the human spirit.

So divine healing is not mental as Christian Science, Unity, and other metaphysical teachers claim. Neither is it only physical as many in the medical world claim. It is spiritual—but only in the sense that it involves faith in the power of God as God's Word proclaims.

I've seen it happen again and again: When people quit trying to contact God with their *mind* and believe they receive in their *heart*, they are healed instantly! You have to believe you receive the things of God by faith—and you believe with your heart (Rom. 10:10)!

With the *Heart* Man Believes

MARK 9:23

23 Jesus said unto him, If thou canst believe, all things are possible to him that believeth.

In chapter 9 of Mark's Gospel, a man came running up to Jesus, telling Him about his son who was possessed by a demon that would throw the boy into fire and water. The disciples had been unable to deliver the boy, so the father begged Jesus, saying, "*. . . if thou canst do any thing, have compassion on us, and help us*" (v. 22).

Jesus replied, "*. . . If thou canst BELIEVE, all things are possible to him that BELIEVETH*" (v. 23).

Notice that Jesus started working immediately on the man's believing, which had to do with his spirit. Jesus turned the father's plea for help around and said, "It's not a matter of what I can do. It's a matter of what you can believe: If thou canst *believe*, all things are possible!"

Your Faith Will Make You Whole

We see this same emphasis on faith repeated again and again in the ministry of Jesus. For example, read the following accounts of Jesus healing the two blind men in Matthew chapter 9, the woman with the issue of blood in Mark chapter 5, and the centurion's servant in Matthew chapter 8.

MATTHEW 9:27-30

27 And when Jesus departed thence, two blind men followed him, crying, and saying, Thou Son of David, have mercy on us.
28 And when he was come into the house, the blind men came to him: and Jesus saith unto them, Believe ye that I am able to do this? They said unto him, Yea, Lord.
29 Then touched he their eyes, saying, According to your faith be it unto you.
30 And their eyes were opened. . . .

MARK 5:25-34

25 And a certain woman, which had an issue of blood twelve years,
26 And had suffered many things of many physicians, and had spent all that she had, and was nothing bettered, but rather grew worse,
27 When she had heard of Jesus, came in the press behind, and touched his garment.
28 For she said, If I may touch but his clothes, I shall be whole.
29 And straightway the fountain of her blood was dried up; and she felt in her body that she was healed of that plague.
30 And Jesus, immediately knowing in himself that virtue had gone out of him, turned him about in the press, and said, Who touched my clothes?
31 And his disciples said unto him, Thou seest the multitude thronging thee, and sayest thou, Who touched me?
32 And he looked round about to see her that had done this thing.
33 But the woman fearing and trembling, knowing what was done in her, came and fell down before him, and told him all the truth.
34 And he said unto her, Daughter, thy faith hath made thee whole; go in peace, and be whole of thy plague.

MATTHEW 8:5-10

5 And when Jesus was entered into Capernaum, there came unto him a centurion, beseeching him,
6 And saying, Lord, my servant lieth at home sick of the palsy, grievously tormented.
7 And Jesus saith unto him, I will come and heal him.
8 The centurion answered and said, Lord, I am not worthy that thou shouldest come under my roof: but speak the word only, and my servant shall be healed.
9 For I am a man under authority, having soldiers under me: and I say to this man, Go, and he goeth; and to another, Come, and he cometh; and to my servant, Do this, and he doeth it.
10 When Jesus heard it, he marvelled, and said to them that followed, Verily I say unto you, I have not found so great faith, no, not in Israel.

What do all these people have in common? They received God's provision of physical healing through their spirit, *because they believed with their heart!*

Questions for Study

1. What is a more accurate translation of the words "griefs" and "sorrows" in Isaiah 53:4?

2. Why don't you need to know anything about Hebrew in order to gain a clear understanding of what Isaiah 53:4 means?

3. Complete this sentence: The human spirit of a lost man or woman is not healed—it's _____.

4. According to Second Corinthians 5:17, when you are in Christ, how many things become new?

5. What does First Peter 2:24 mean?

6. What is the only sense in which divine healing could be called spiritual healing?

7. How does man heal?

8. How does God heal?

9. What happens when people quit trying to contact God with their mind and believe they receive in their heart?

10. What do the two blind men in Matthew 9, the woman with the issue of blood in Mark 5, and the centurion's servant in Matthew 8 have in common?

Chapter 10

Walk in the Light of God's Word

I've said it before, but it bears repeating: *Jesus is the will of God in action! If you want to see God work, look at Jesus; if you want to hear God talk, listen to Jesus.*

JOHN 14:9
9 Jesus saith unto him [Philip] **. . . he that hath seen me hath seen the Father. . . .**

Well, what do we see Jesus doing in His earthly ministry? We see Him going about *doing good* and *healing* (Acts 10:38). So if Jesus is the will of God in action, then it must be the will of God to heal.

Healing *Is* God's Will

Healing has always been in God's plan of redemption. But many people don't receive their healing because of unbelief.

As we saw in the previous chapter, healing is no longer a matter of what God can do; it's a matter of what we can believe. We looked at Mark chapter 9 and the man who came to Jesus, telling him about his demon-possessed son who threw himself into fire and water. The disciples had been unable to deliver the man's son.

The father begged Jesus, ". . . if thou canst do any thing, have compassion on us, and help us" (v. 22). Remember what Jesus replied: ". . . *If thou canst believe, all things are possible to him that believeth*" (v. 23). Jesus immediately started working on the man's believing, which had to do with his spirit. Jesus turned his plea for help around and said, "It's not a matter of what I can do; it's a matter of what you can believe."

We see this emphasis on faith repeated again and again in the ministry of Jesus. We looked at three specific examples in the previous chapter: the healing of the two blind men in Matthew 9, the healing of the woman with the issue of blood in Mark 5, and the healing of the centurion's servant in Matthew 8. These people received healing through their spirits, because they believed with their hearts!

Notice what the psalmist of old said in Psalm 107:

PSALM 107:20
20 He sent his word, and healed them, and delivered them from their destructions.

The word that God sent under the Old Covenant was spoken by the prophets. But the word that God sent under the New Covenant was the Lord Jesus Christ, the Word of God (John 1:1,14). God sent His Word—the Living Word—and healed us.

Therefore, in the mind of God, we're already healed! He's already sent His Word and healed us.

We're Already Healed!

God has given us the written Word so that we'll know what the Living Word has done for us. And we know that the Living Word healed us: He took our infirmities and bare our sicknesses; and by His stripes we *were* healed (Ps. 107:20; Matt. 8:17; 1 Peter 2:24).

Well, "were" is past tense. That means we're already healed! (You have to get your believing in the right tense for it to work for you!)

Now God will often let another person believe for you when you don't know the Word or you're still in the babyhood stage of Christianity. He will meet you on a lower level of faith.

Once we receive light from the Word concerning God's will to heal, He expects us to walk in that light. God expects mature believers to walk in the light of what they know. That's why it's the most difficult thing in the world for some Christians to get healed—because they already have light concerning healing, and God expects them to walk in that light, but they're not!

God's Word Is a Seed

God's Word contains all you need for a successful Christian life. But it won't work for you if you just place the Bible on your coffee table. God's Word will never produce for you until you plant it in your heart and cultivate it.

1 CORINTHIANS 3:6-9
6 I [Paul] have planted, Apollos watered; but God gave the increase.
7 So then neither is he that planteth any thing, neither he that watereth; but God that giveth the increase.
8 Now he that planteth and he that watereth are one: and every man shall receive his own reward according to his own labour.
9 For we are labourers together with God: ye are God's husbandry, ye are God's building.

The word "husbandry" in verse 9 is a little blind to us. The Greek translation of this phrase is "ye are God's *tillage*." That might still be a little blind to some people. Other versions of the Bible translate "husbandry" as *farm* or *garden*. So Paul was really saying that the Church at Corinth was God's garden.

Well, that's true concerning the Church today; we are God's garden or farm. A gardener or farmer tills the soil; that's why Paul said, "I planted." But the seed that Paul planted (in the hearts of the Corinthians) was the Word of God.

In Luke 8:5-18, Jesus told the parable of the sower, and in explaining it to His disciples He said, "*. . . The seed is the word of God*" (v. 11). Let's take a closer look at this parable as it is recorded in the Gospel of Mark because it gives a little more detail than Luke's account.

MARK 4:3-8
3 Hearken; Behold, there went out a sower to sow:
4 And it came to pass, as he sowed, some fell by the way side, and the fowls of the air came and devoured it up.
5 And some fell on stony ground, where it had not much earth; and immediately it sprang up, because it had no depth of earth:
6 But when the sun was up, it was scorched; and because it had no root, it withered away.
7 And some fell among thorns, and the thorns grew up, and choked it, and it yielded no fruit.
8 And other fell on good ground, and did yield fruit that sprang up and increased; and brought forth, some thirty, and some sixty, and some an hundred.

You see, the different types of ground didn't all bring forth a hundredfold—not even the good ground (v. 8). I guess that was the best they could do. But, thank God, some did bring forth a hundredfold! It's not up to God to decide which type of ground you're going to be. It's up to *you*.

I remember preaching in a certain place years ago; it seemed like my preaching wasn't doing much good. So I started doing a little extra praying and fasting. Then one day the Lord said to me: "I told you ahead of time that only one out of four people is going to catch on to what you're saying."

I said, "What?"

The Lord said, "I told you ahead of time that only one out of four will understand what you're saying. And of the one-fourth who get it, only a third of them will bring forth full fruit, or a hundredfold."

Well, I didn't catch on right away to what He was saying, so I asked, "What are You talking about?"

Then the Lord asked me a question: "Don't you remember the parable of the sower?"

"Yes," I said, "I remember that."

Then the Lord explained that parable to me, saying, "The sower went forth to sow. Some seed fell by the wayside and the fowls of the air devoured it. Those are the one-fourth who heard the Word but didn't understand it, and the devil came and stole it away from them. Of course, they had to permit that because the devil can't steal from you unless you let him (1 Peter 5:8).

"Some seed fell on stony ground, and it sprung up right away. Did you ever see those folks who looked as though they were going to become spiritual 'giants' overnight? They're responding to the Word so well, but they don't have any depth. They don't have any root. So when the sun rises and beats upon them, the Word in their hearts just dies and withers away. Then they disappear and you wonder where they went. That makes two-fourths who didn't get it."

Then the Lord said, "Some seed fell among the thorns and the thistles—the cares of this life.

Many people become too concerned with the cares of life. That care chokes out the seed, and it dies without producing any results. So that accounts for the three out of four who didn't get it."

But, thank God, some seed fell on good ground and brought forth, some thirtyfold, some sixtyfold, and some a hundredfold!

I knew the parable of the sower, but I never had seen it that way before. What the Lord said really surprised me, but it also encouraged me. I found out that I was doing better than I had thought!

It's Your Responsibility To Walk In the Light of the Word

Jesus told us ahead of time that not everyone would walk in the light of the Word (Mark 4:3-8). But what most people don't realize is that what you do with the Word is up to *you*, the hearer.

At the last church I pastored, there was a fellow who wasn't a member of our church, but he visited our church regularly. One day he said to me, "I would sure hate to be in your shoes."

Well, I looked down at my shoes, because I didn't know if he was talking about the pair of shoes I had on.

So I asked him, "What do you mean you'd 'hate to be in my shoes'? Are you talking about the shoes on my feet? Or do you mean you'd hate to be in my place—married to the woman I'm married to or driving the car I'm driving? What do you mean by that statement?"

Then a really serious look came on the man's face and he said, "Why, don't you know that you'll have to give an account to God for everything you preach and teach?"

I said, "Don't you know that *you're* going to have to give an account to God for everything that I preach and teach?"

He said, "What! Me!"

I said, "Yes! And I'll prove it to you by the Word." I went over the parable of the sower with him. Then I asked him, "Did you notice that in all the time Jesus spent telling that story He only mentioned the *sower* once? Jesus never said anything about the sower's responsibility. He spent all of His time talking about the *hearer*. He wound up talking about the hearer's responsibility by saying, *'Take heed therefore how ye hear . . .'"* (Luke 8:18). You see, it makes all the difference in the world how you hear!

Of course, ministers are responsible for what they preach and teach, but where does the greater responsibility lie? With the hearer!

Take Heed How You Hear

Several years ago, my wife took responsibility for how she heard when her doctor discovered a blockage in her heart. The doctor wanted to run further tests to see whether he could treat it with medication or if he would have to perform surgery.

So my wife started listening to my "Healing Scriptures" audiotape. She listened to it almost constantly, and she meditated on the Word day in and day out. In other words, she was taking heed how she heard. She always gets up before I do. When I woke up in the morning, I saw the light on in the bathroom, and I heard the tape playing.

She spent hours on end just listening to the Word. (I don't mean hours at one time, but when you add up the time.) Then the Holy Ghost took certain verses and quickened them to her. My wife began to confess those scriptures, and that blockage just disappeared! Her doctor told us, "This is the first miracle I've ever seen. I want you to know there is nothing wrong with your heart. Your heart is perfect in every way. You don't need medication, and you don't need any surgery. Your heart is perfect, and you can tell people your doctor said so!"

My wife took heed how she heard and it produced healing for her. Jesus said, *"Take heed therefore how ye hear . . ."* (Luke 8:18). Well, how did my wife hear? The answer is found in Romans 10:17.

ROMANS 10:17
17 So then faith cometh by HEARING, AND HEARING by the word of God.

This verse is talking about hearing, isn't it? Does faith come by hearing one time? No, faith comes by hearing and hearing and hearing. My wife kept hearing, and she received her healing.

A few years after my wife received her healing, she found out that a friend of hers also had a critical condition that could prove to be fatal. In talking with her, my wife asked, "Do you have Brother Hagin's 'Healing Scriptures' tape?"

Her friend said, "Yes, I believe I do have it." But when my wife asked her if she was listening to it, her friend said, "Oh, I've heard it. I listened to it years ago."

Romans 10:17 doesn't say, "So then faith comes from having *heard*." No. It says that faith comes by *hearing*. Then you have to take heed how you hear.

Well, my wife told her friend what she had done, but the woman didn't catch on to what my wife was saying. That woman esteemed the Word lightly, so it never produced healing in her life. My wife esteemed the Word highly, and it produced highly in her life!

An Elder's Story

In September 1954, I was holding a three-week revival in a Foursquare church in California. The pastor's father-in-law would come regularly and sit in on the day services. He was an elderly gentleman—about eighty-two years old.

When we got into the third week of the meeting, this man came up to me after the morning service and asked, "Brother Hagin, may I speak to you?"

I said, "Yes." And he told me his story.

He said, "I came to California from Indiana in 1923. I had a physical condition that was terminal. The doctors told me that if I'd move out West where the winters weren't as severe, I might live another two years. So I packed up— lock, stock, and barrel—and moved my family to Los Angeles, California.

"That was the year Mrs. Aimee Semple McPherson built the 5,000-seat Angelus Temple in Los Angeles. Someone told me about her healing meetings, and I went. Of course, I was

desperate, because the doctors had said nothing more could be done for me.

"So I got in Mrs. McPherson's healing line and was healed by the power of God! Then I found out that I wasn't saved. I had always been a good church member, active in church work, and had just supposed that I already was a Christian. But I got saved and baptized with the Holy Ghost at her meeting too.

"I went to church there every week afterward and continued to hear the Word taught until we moved to northern California in 1933. Then in 1938 I developed a hernia. I said to my wife, 'I know all I have to do is have Mrs. McPherson lay hands on me, and that rupture will disappear.'

"While I was making plans to go to Los Angeles, I developed another rupture. Now I had a *double* hernia. When I did get back to the Angelus Temple, folks were beginning to come from everywhere for the daily healing meetings. It took me five days to get in the line, but finally Mrs. McPherson ministered to me—and I didn't get a thing!"

'Aimee's Lost It'

"I thought, *Mrs. McPherson didn't have it tonight. If she had it like she did fifteen years ago, I would have gotten healed. But she didn't have it. So I'll just have to wait here until she gets it.*

"I stayed another five days with some kinfolks. That's how long it took me to get back in the healing line again. When she laid hands on me the second time, I didn't get a thing.

"My relatives asked me, 'Well, did you get healed?'

"I said, 'No. Whatever Mrs. McPherson had, she lost it. I went through her line twice. I guess she doesn't have it anymore.'"

'The Evangelists Don't Have It Either'

"Brother Hagin, I carried my double hernia ten more years, from 1938 to 1948. Then while I was in the San Joaquin Valley, I happened to pick up a paper and noticed that some fellow was putting up a tent in Stockton. The ad said, 'Bring the blind, see the lame walk,' and so on. Well, all I had to do was get to Stockton!

"I went to this evangelist's meeting several times. He laid hands on me, but I didn't get a thing. I finally decided, *He doesn't have what he claims to have. If he had what Mrs. McPherson had—well, she had it, but she lost it—then I would have been healed!*

"Not too long after that, I saw in the paper that another fellow was holding a tent meeting in Sacramento. I knew all I had to do was get over to those meetings. So this other evangelist in Sacramento laid hands on me too, and I came away with both of my hernias. I said, '*He* doesn't have it either.'"

Wasted Time

"I wound up going to several other meetings to be prayed for, and every time I'd go away saying, 'They don't have it!' Then last year in Santa Cruz, a famous prophet and evangelist was scheduled to preach at our church's campmeeting. I went to the meeting, got in his healing line, and without my ever telling him a word, he told me exactly what was wrong with me by the word of knowledge. But I didn't get healed.

"I went away once more saying, 'This brother doesn't have it. If he'd had what Mrs. McPherson had, I'd have gotten healed. Of course, *she* had it—but she lost it.'

"Then this year, Brother Hagin, *you* were advertised to preach at our campmeeting. I had heard about the vision you had of Jesus and how He appeared unto you, because it was published all through the church. I knew all I had to do was get to Santa Cruz and get in your healing line.

"I don't know how many times you laid hands on me in that campmeeting and later here in my son's church. But I wasn't healed. I said, 'I guess *Brother Hagin* doesn't have it. If he had what *Mrs. McPherson* had back in '23—of course, now she's lost it—I'd have gotten healed.'"

Then this elderly man said to me, "But, you know, Brother Hagin, since I've been sitting here in these day services listening to you, I'm beginning to see something."

"What?" I asked.

"I'm beginning to see that God requires something of me."

I said, "Yes, brother. I don't mind telling you, you're wasting your time getting in healing lines. You've wasted sixteen years trying to get healed on someone else's faith. Why, instead of having to be prayed for, you ought to be out praying for the sick yourself. No, brother, you're going to have to get healed on your own faith!"

You Have a Part To Play

You see, I was teaching on the subjects "How To Put Your Faith To Work" and "How To Confess With Your Mouth and Believe in Your Heart" in those daytime sessions. By sitting in on the services, that gentleman had begun to learn that *he* had a part to play.

That was in September 1954. In July 1955, ten months later, I went up to the Old Oak Ranch in the Sonora Mountains to preach for some Foursquare churches in that district. And one of the first fellows I saw was this elderly man. He was now eighty-three.

He waved at me from a distance and called, "Brother Hagin, Brother Hagin!" I waited for him to catch up with me.

Here he came running—at eighty-three! He threw his arms around me and hugged me. "Brother Hagin," he shouted, jumping up and down, "I'm completely healed! Both of my hernias have disappeared. I carried them around all those years, but now they're gone—and I got healed on my own faith!

"Not only that," he said, "but I'm doing just what you said. I'm eighty-three and retired, you know. So I'm out visiting the sick every day, praying for them and getting them healed!"

Praise God! That man was healed of his terminal illness back in 1923 through Aimee Semple McPherson's ministry because he was new in the faith. But years later when he developed those two hernias, something was required of *him*. God was requiring him to exercise his own faith.

You Have To Exercise Your Own Faith

When I minister healing, I lay hands on the sick in obedience to the spiritual law of "contact and transmission"—the contact of my hands transmits God's healing power into their bodies to undo that which Satan has wrought and to affect in them a healing and a cure (Mark 16:18; Acts 19:11,12).

Once I'm conscious that God's healing power has gone into them, I say, "There it is." That's as far as I can take people. That's where my responsibility ends and theirs begins.

You see, divine healing has to be appropriated by faith. You may be able to receive it through another person's faith for a while. But sooner or later you'll have to learn to exercise your own faith.

The Word of God is clear—God's will is healing. Now it's time to walk in the light of the Word you've received.

Questions for Study

1. What do we see Jesus doing in His earthly ministry?

   _____

   _____

2. If Jesus is the will of God in action, what does that tell us about healing?

   _____

   _____

3. What does Psalm 107:20 say about healing?

   _____

   _____

4. Under the Old Covenant, the word that God sent was spoken by whom?

   _____

   _____

5. Why has God given us the written Word?

   _____

   _____

6. When will God let another person believe for your healing?

   _____

   _____

7. What does God expect mature believers to do?

   _____

   _____

8. Why is it the most difficult thing in the world for some Christians to get healed?

   _____

   _____

9. What is the spiritual law of contact and transmission?

   _____

   _____

10. How is divine healing appropriated?

    _____

    _____

Chapter 11

Knowing and Acting on God's Word

By putting God's anointed Word in your heart, you can learn to walk in freedom in every area of your life. When you believe and act upon God's anointed Word, the anointing will break the yoke of bondage and set you free in every area of your life!

ISAIAH 10:27
27 . . . the yoke shall be destroyed because of the anointing.

We often hear it said that it's the anointing that breaks every yoke. But what is a "yoke" in present-day application? A "yoke" is *anything that binds people*. For example, a yoke can be sin, sickness or disease, poverty, or oppression by evil spirits. But, thank God, the yoke shall be destroyed because of the anointing!

My Testimony of Healing

I was sickly until I was seventeen years old. I didn't grow up normally because for the first sixteen years of my life, I couldn't run and play like other children. I played very limitedly because I had a deformed heart and an incurable blood disease. The blood disease made my blood pale orange in color instead of red, and there were other complications. I never had a normal childhood, and about four months before my sixteenth birthday, I became totally bedfast.

Several doctors had been called in on my case. The great Mayo Clinic in Rochester, Minnesota, hailed one of the doctors on my case as one of the best surgeons in the world. This doctor said that no one in my condition in the history of medical science had ever lived past the age of sixteen.

But, thank God for the Bible, which is God's holy written Word. *The Word is anointed!* It's filled with God's power, and God's anointed Word destroys every yoke of bondage, including the yoke of sickness and disease. That's how I was raised up off the bed of sickness—by acting on God's anointed Word.

I had read the Bible as a young Baptist boy, but I didn't know much about acting on the Word. For example, I knew that the Holy Spirit lived inside me. But I didn't know at first that I was supposed *to listen* to Him or that He would guide me to act on God's Word.

JOHN 16:13
13 Howbeit when he, the Spirit of truth, is come, he will GUIDE YOU INTO ALL TRUTH: for he shall not speak of himself; but whatsoever he shall hear, that shall he speak: and he will shew you things to come.

I've thought about it many times since then that if I had listened to the Holy Spirit sooner, I would not have stayed bedfast for those sixteen months. But I was so busy trying to get someone to help me that I failed to listen to the Holy Spirit on the inside of me. That's where we miss it so many times. Most of us are looking for something in the natural to help us. But if you are saved, the Holy Spirit abides in your spirit, and the Bible says He'll guide you into all truth. God's Word is truth (John 17:17).

'It's All in the Book'

During the time I was bedfast, the Holy Spirit kept trying to tell me I could be healed. Finally one day, I heard something on the inside of me—that still, small voice—say, "You don't have to die at this early age. You can be healed." Well, if I could be healed, I wanted to know *how*. I knew medical science couldn't do anything for me. So I asked the Lord, "*How* can I be healed?" And that same inward voice said, "It's all in the Book."

When I heard the words, "It's all in the Book," I knew the Holy Spirit was talking about the Bible, so I began to diligently study the Bible day and night. When I read Mark 11:23 and 24, those words were branded on my spirit like a branding iron brands cattle.

MARK 11:23,24

23 For verily I [Jesus] say unto you, That whosoever shall say unto this mountain, Be thou removed, and be thou cast into the sea; and shall not doubt in his heart, but shall believe that those things which he saith shall come to pass; he shall have whatsoever he saith.

24 Therefore I say unto you, What things soever ye desire [and that includes healing], when ye pray, believe that ye receive them, and ye shall have them.

Those words, *". . . What things soever ye desire, when ye pray, believe that ye receive them, and ye shall have them"* (v. 24), became indelibly imprinted on my heart. You see, the greatest desire of my heart was to be healed. More than sixty-five years ago, as I acted on God's anointed Word, His Word brought healing to my body. And I've been healed ever since!

We've Already Been Redeemed From Sickness!

Healing belongs to us as believers. At the time I was healed, I didn't know about our redemption from sickness and disease. I didn't know about Isaiah 53:4 and 5 and other scriptures about Christ's redemptive work.

ISAIAH 53:4,5

4 Surely he [Jesus] hath borne our griefs, and carried our sorrows [the original Hebrew says He bore our sicknesses and carried our pains]**: yet we did esteem him stricken, smitten of God, and afflicted.**

5 But he was wounded for our transgressions, he was bruised for our iniquities: the chastisement of our peace was upon him; and with his stripes we are healed.

MATTHEW 8:17

17 That it might be fulfilled which was spoken by Esaias [Isaiah] the prophet, saying, Himself [Jesus] took our infirmities, and bare our sicknesses.

1 PETER 2:24

24 Who his own self [Jesus] bare our sins in his own body on the tree, that we, being dead to sins, should live unto righteousness: by whose stripes ye were healed.

Many times, this is where folks miss it. They say, "I know God promised to heal me, but He hasn't done it *yet*." This causes folks to become confused.

But God didn't promise to heal them *someday*. He said in His Word that they are healed *now*!

To say that God has promised to heal us is like an unsaved person saying, "I know God has promised to save me." No. God didn't *promise* to save the sinner. The Word says that salvation *belongs to every unsaved person right now*! Second Corinthians 5:19 says, *". . . God was in Christ, reconciling the world unto himself, not imputing their trespasses unto them. . . ."* Salvation is a gift. It was paid for by Jesus Christ. It belongs to us.

Healing belongs to us too! And receiving healing, just like receiving salvation, is simply a matter of appropriating what already belongs to us because of Christ's redemptive work.

Someone might say, "I've read all those wonderful promises in the Word." But these scriptures on healing that we just read are not really promises; they are *statements of fact*. Remember, in the mind of God, you're already healed. God has already healed you because He laid sickness and disease on Jesus. Jesus has already borne sickness and disease for you. You need not bear what Jesus already bore for you.

When Isaiah wrote about Jesus' redemptive work, *"Surely he hath borne our griefs, and carried our sorrows . . ."* (Isa. 53:4), he was prophesying about the future. He was looking forward in time to the Cross. Some people say that verse was only prophesying concerning salvation. However, we know the words "griefs" and "sorrows" are literally translated from the Hebrew as "sickness" and "pain." So our redemption included both remission of sin and physical healing.

When Peter later wrote about Jesus' redemptive work, *"Who his own self bare our sins in his own body on the tree . . . by whose stripes ye were healed"* (1 Peter 2:24), he was looking back in time to the Cross.

Peter wrote, *". . . by whose stripes ye WERE healed."* Since you *were* healed, you *are* healed. In other words, you're not *going to be* healed. You *are* healed! And as you stand in faith on God's Word, your body has to come in line with God's Word, and every symptom has to go!

Someone might say, "I just believe God is going to heal me *sometime*." Well, that's not agreeing with God. In fact, to say that is really taking sides *against* God because God and His Word are one. God's Word is God speaking to us, and God's Word says we *were* healed (1 Peter 2:24)!

Feed Your Spirit Continually

Some people are always wanting God to speak to them, but if they'd get in the Bible and read it and meditate on it, they'd find that God is speaking to them from every page. They're always looking for some "new" revelation, yet they haven't mastered walking in the light of what they already know. But when you walk in the light of what you know, more light will be given to you. You see, it's the truth of God's anointed Word, not some "new" revelation, that sets people free and destroys every yoke of bondage.

Sometimes when I've tried to read scriptures to people on healing, they've said, "Oh, I've already heard that." That's like a man sitting down at the table to eat, but when a big T-bone steak is put on his plate, he says, "No thanks. I've had T-bone steak before"! Just because you ate a T-bone steak one time doesn't mean you're never going to eat one again!

MATTHEW 4:4
4 . . . Man shall not live by bread alone, but by every word that proceedeth out of the mouth of God.

What is this verse saying? It's saying that what natural food is to your body, the Word of God is to your spirit. The Word of God is "food" or nourishment, for your spirit. Just because you ate a certain kind of natural food one time doesn't mean you're never going to eat it again. No, you'll come right back to the table and eat the same kinds of food again and again.

The Truth Will Set You Free!

When it comes to spiritual things, a preacher can teach on faith and healing and sometimes people say, "Oh, I've heard that before." But in much the same way that we eat the same kind of natural food again and again, we need to come right back to God's table and eat *His* food—the Word of God—again and again.

ROMANS 10:17
17 So then faith cometh by hearing, and hearing by the word of God.

Faith comes by *hearing* and *hearing* the Word of God. In other words, faith doesn't come by hearing it just once or even by hearing it occasionally. The Word of God is anointed and if you get that Word in your heart by hearing it again and again, the anointing will set you free.

JOHN 8:32
32 And ye shall KNOW the truth, and the truth shall make you free.

The truth sets you free. We know that God's Word is truth (John 17:17). The truth of the anointed Word will set you free, but the truth can't set you free until you *know* the truth. The way you know the truth is by putting it in your heart—in your spirit. And the way you do that is by hearing the Word continually.

As I shared in a previous chapter, several years ago, my wife Oretha became physically weak and just kept getting weaker. When she went to have a medical exam, her doctor discovered a blockage in one side of her heart and immediately ordered more tests. He also told her not to exert herself physically at all. So she spent time in the Word constantly, putting God's medicine—His Word—in her spirit. She listened to my tape called "Healing Scriptures" almost constantly.

Oretha was scheduled to go back to the doctor for more tests to see whether she would need surgery or if medication alone could help her. One evening before her return visit to the doctor, she was meditating on the Word, thinking about the goodness of God, when she felt something like two hands reach down into her heart and take something out.

She went back to the same doctor for more tests, and he couldn't find a thing wrong with her heart! He said the blockage was gone and that her heart was perfectly normal! Her doctor was a Christian, and he said that was the first miracle of that sort he had ever seen. He had seen other people helped through both prayer and medicine, but he had never seen a miracle like hers. What had happened? She just kept putting that Word in her spirit, and God healed her through His anointed Word.

You Must Do Your Part

Healing belongs to us, but most folks miss it because they think, *If healing belongs to me, why don't I have it?* In other words, they think the blessings of God are just going to automatically fall on them like ripe cherries fall off a tree. But that's not true. The blessings of God must be *appropriated* by faith in God's written Word. In other words, we must receive by faith the blessings that God has already provided for us in His Word.

The same is true with salvation. For example, have you ever stopped to think about the fact that the New Birth, the remission of sin, belongs to the worst sinner, just as much as it belongs to the Christian? The remission of sin belongs to people in jail or prison—even those who are on "death row"—just as much as it belongs to the most faithful churchgoer. Why? Because the Bible says, *"For God so loved THE WORLD, that he gave his only begotten Son, that WHOSOEVER believeth in him should not perish, but have everlasting life"* (John 3:16).

Jesus paid for salvation for every man, woman, boy, and girl who would ever live on this earth. But people must believe on Jesus and receive Him as their own Savior before salvation can benefit them.

So, you see, salvation belongs to the sinner. Then why doesn't every sinner get saved? It's either because no one has shared the Gospel with him, so he doesn't know about salvation, or because someone has told him about salvation, but he didn't believe it or accept it.

The same thing is true with healing. One reason many Christians haven't received healing is they haven't heard the Word, and they don't know healing belongs to them. They thought they had to stay sick. But healing still belongs to them. There are other reasons Christians don't get healed as well, but the point is, healing belongs to them.

We know it's the anointing that destroys every yoke of sickness and disease. But actually, the anointing is released by *acting* on God's anointed Word—that is, by *believing* it and *applying* it to your own life.

It's a Done Deal!

Years ago a crippled woman who hadn't walked in four years attended a meeting I held. She was seventy-two years old and doctors said she would never walk another step. I read Matthew 8:17 and First Peter 2:24 to her. She said, "Yes, I know those scriptures, and I believe them."

I asked her to read aloud the last part of First Peter 2:24, and she read, *". . . by whose stripes ye were healed."* I said, "Read it again," and she did. Then I asked her, "Is 'were' past tense, present tense, or future tense?"

She looked at me in amazement, and I could see that the light had suddenly dawned on her. She said, "Why, it's past tense. And if we *were* healed, then I *was* healed."

"That's right," I encouraged her. Then I said, "You're still sitting there crippled. You haven't moved a bit. You need to start believing that you *were* healed when the stripes were laid on Jesus. If you believe that, then begin to say, 'If I *was* healed, then I *am* healed.' Start believing you *are* healed *now*."

I talked to this crippled woman about what the Word says, and just kept quoting the Word to her on healing. After about ten minutes, she was leaping and walking and praising God! Some people in that church said, "That Hagin fellow healed a crippled woman in church the other night." But I didn't do any such thing! I can't heal anyone. *Jesus* purchased her healing more than 2,000 years ago. She just found out about it that night!

God's anointed Word will work for you, too, and set you free from every yoke of bondage—sin, sickness or disease, poverty, or anything else the devil tries to bring against you. But you must *act* on God's Word by agreeing with it. You must believe it and feed upon it. That's how you get it into your heart or spirit. As God's Word becomes a part of you, the anointing will deliver you and bring freedom to every area of your life.

70

Questions for Study

1. When will the anointing break the yoke of bondage and set you free in every area of your life?
   _____
   _____

2. What is a yoke in present-day application?
   _____
   _____

3. According to John 16:13, what are three ways in which the Holy Spirit helps believers?
   _____
   _____

4. What similarities are there between salvation and healing?
   _____
   _____

5. The scriptures on healing are not really promises. What are they?
   _____
   _____

6. Some people are always looking for some "new" revelation, yet they haven't mastered walking in the light of what they already know. When will more light be given to them?
   _____
   _____

7. In what way is natural food similar to the Word of God?
   _____
   _____

8. When will the truth of the anointed Word set you free?
   _____
   _____

9. Does the remission of sins belong to people in jail or prison? Why or why not?
   _____
   _____

10. List two reasons why many sick Christians don't get healed.
    _____
    _____

Chapter 12

There's Healing Power in the Name of Jesus!

The Name of Jesus belongs to you as a Christian, and you have a right to use that Name. But you need to *know* the power and the authority that's in Jesus' Name, and you must learn to *exercise* that authority.

JOHN 14:12-14
12 Verily, verily, I [Jesus] **say unto you, He that believeth on me, the works that I do shall he do also; and greater works than these shall he do; because I go unto my Father.**
13 **And whatsoever ye shall ask in my name, that will I do, that the Father may be glorified in the Son.**
14 **If ye shall ask any thing in my name, I will do it.**

Many times, when we just sort of "skim" over the Word of God, we miss the impact of what the Word is saying. For example, many people believe that John 14:12-14 is a reference to the subject of prayer. However, a closer examination of this passage will reveal that it is really referring to the believer's right to exercise spiritual authority in the Name of Jesus.

Make a Demand in the Name of Jesus

According to *Strong's Exhaustive Concordance*, the meaning of the Greek word "ask" in John 14:13,14 implies *a demand of something due*. Jesus told the disciples, *"If ye shall ASK* [demand] *any thing IN MY NAME, I WILL DO IT"* (John 14:14). Jesus was not talking about prayer here; He was talking about using His Name as a basis for authority.

In the Early Church, healing was used as a means of advertising the Gospel as well as a means of blessing and helping people. The Apostle Peter knew that there is power in the Name of Jesus. Peter used the authority in that Name to command sickness and disease to go.

ACTS 3:1-16
1 **Now Peter and John went up together into the temple at the hour of prayer, being the ninth hour.**
2 **And a certain man lame from his mother's womb was carried, whom they laid daily at the gate of the** temple which is called Beautiful, to ask alms of them that entered into the temple;
3 **Who seeing Peter and John about to go into the temple asked an alms.**
4 **And Peter, fastening his eyes upon him with John, said, Look on us.**
5 **And he gave heed unto them, expecting to receive something of them.**
6 **Then Peter said, Silver and gold have I none; but such as I have give I thee: IN THE NAME OF JESUS CHRIST of Nazareth rise up and walk.**
7 **And he took him by the right hand, and lifted him up: and immediately his feet and ankle bones received strength.**
8 **And he leaping up stood, and walked, and entered with them into the temple, walking, and leaping, and praising God.**
9 **And all the people saw him walking and praising God:**
10 **And they knew that it was he which sat for alms at the Beautiful gate of the temple: and they were filled with wonder and amazement at that which had happened unto him.**
11 **And as the lame man which was healed held Peter and John, all the people ran together unto them in the porch that is called Solomon's, greatly wondering.**
12 **And when Peter saw it, he answered unto the people, Ye men of Israel, why marvel ye at this? or why look ye so earnestly on us, as though by our own power or holiness we had made this man to walk?**
13 **The God of Abraham, and of Isaac, and of Jacob, the God of our fathers, hath glorified his Son Jesus; whom ye delivered up, and denied him in the presence of Pilate, when he was determined to let him go.**
14 **But ye denied the Holy One and the Just, and desired a murderer to be granted unto you;**
15 **And killed the Prince of life, whom God hath raised from the dead; whereof we are witnesses.**
16 **And his name through faith in his name hath made this man strong, whom ye see and know: yea, the faith which is by him hath given him this perfect soundness in the presence of you all.**

Peter didn't demand anything of *God* when he commanded, *". . . In the name of Jesus Christ of Nazareth rise up and walk"* (v. 6). You see, God never made that man crippled to begin with—Satan did. Peter used the Name of Jesus to set the crippled man free from the bondage of Satan.

Peter demanded that the man arise and walk in Jesus' Name, because Jesus said, "Whatever you demand in My Name, I will do!"

When the man was healed, the crowd thought that Peter and John had healed him. If people aren't careful, they will look to man to heal them. Later in Acts 3:16, Peter told the people exactly how the crippled man had been made whole. He said, *"And HIS* [Jesus'] *NAME through faith in HIS NAME hath made this man strong, whom ye see and know: yea, the faith which is by him hath given him this perfect soundness. . . ."* You see, it is that Name—the Name of Jesus—which guarantees the answer!

The Name of Jesus Belongs to You!

As Christians, the Name of Jesus belongs to us. Yet many times, that Name doesn't mean as much to believers as it should because their thinking is wrong. If your thinking is wrong, your believing will be wrong; and if your believing is wrong, then what you say will be wrong too. It all goes back to your thinking. You've got to get your thinking straightened out in order for the Name of Jesus to mean what it should mean to you.

The Bible says, *". . . faith cometh by hearing, and hearing by the word of God"* (Rom. 10:17). You've got to have *faith* in the Name of Jesus before that Name will produce results for you. When your faith in the Name of Jesus increases, then the results will increase!

Some Christians think of the Name of Jesus in the same way they think of a good luck charm. They have about as much faith in the Name of Jesus as they have in a rabbit's foot! They say, "Maybe it will work," or "I hope something good comes out of it." As long as they just *try* the Name of Jesus as though it's some sort of good luck charm—nothing will happen for them, unless God in His mercy intervenes on their behalf and does something for them in spite of themselves.

Using the Name of Jesus To Obtain Healing

The Name of Jesus belongs to you as a Christian, and you have a right to use that Name. When sickness or disease tries to attack you, you can command it to leave your body. That's how I've been able to live for more than sixty-five years now without having a headache. I didn't say symptoms of a headache never tried to attack me. I said I haven't had a headache in more than sixty-five years. When a symptom came, I demanded it to leave in Jesus' Name, and it left!

If sickness or disease comes to you, instead of accepting it and talking about your troubles, say, "In the Name of Jesus Christ of Nazareth, leave my body!" And the sickness or disease must go! You may say, "I tried that, and it didn't work." Using the Name of Jesus doesn't work by *trying* it; it works by *doing* it! Your spirit man—the real you on the inside—is the ruler of your body. In other words, you are the ruler, or the caretaker of your own body. You are the one who must exercise dominion over it—not someone else.

I once read about a man who was the caretaker of some landscaped property. After repeated efforts to stop people from walking on the grass, this caretaker posted a sign that read: "Gentlemen *will not*, and others *must not* trespass on this property." You see, you—not someone else—are the caretaker of your physical body, and you have a right to forbid Satan to trespass against your body with sickness or disease!

The Apostle Paul said, *"But I keep under my body, and bring it into subjection: lest that by any means, when I have preached to others, I myself should be a castaway"* (1 Cor. 9:27). To bring something into subjection means to rule over something or to take authority over something.

I like what Smith Wigglesworth said: "If someone asks, 'How is Smith Wigglesworth feeling today?' I tell him, 'I never *ask* Smith Wigglesworth how he feels; I *tell* him how he feels!'"

That's right in line with what Paul said: *"I bring my body into subjection."* Some Christians don't bring their bodies into subjection— they are body-ruled. That's what it means to be *carnal.* Yet every Christian has the ability to bring his or her body into subjection, as Paul did. Just because Paul was an apostle, doesn't mean he was any more saved than you are; he didn't have any more authority over his body than you do over yours. But Paul *exercised* his authority. *He* brought his body into subjection.

ROMANS 12:1
1 **I beseech you therefore, brethren, by the mercies of God, that ye present your bodies a living sacrifice, holy, acceptable unto God, which is your reasonable service.**

Paul addressed the Book of Romans to believers. Romans 1:7 says, *"To all that be in Rome, beloved of God, called to be saints. . . ."* So Romans 12:1 applies to all the beloved of God, called to be saints—whether they are in Rome or in your own hometown. Paul admonished all believers: *". . . present your bodies a living sacrifice . . . which is your reasonable service"* (v. 1). One translation says, "which is your spiritual service." Paul said presenting your body to God as a living sacrifice is your spiritual service, and that applies to *every* believer.

You are the ruler of your own body. If you weren't the ruler of your own body, then you couldn't bring it into subjection, and you couldn't present it to God as a living sacrifice according to Romans 12:1. You wouldn't be able to take authority over any sickness or disease that might try to harm you. But you *are* the ruler of your own body, and, thank God, you have a right to freedom from pain, sickness, and disease in the Name of Jesus! But you must exercise the authority which belongs to you *in that Name.*

When you take authority over sickness or disease in your body and command it to leave in Jesus' Name, you are demanding something due you: freedom from whatever it is that has attacked your body. John 14:14 says, *"If ye shall ask* [or demand] *any thing in my name, I will do it."* You're not demanding anything of God; you're demanding something of demon forces because sickness and disease come from the devil, not from God.

Jesus told the disciples to pray, *". . . Thy will be done in earth, as it is in heaven"* (Matt. 6:10).

There isn't any sickness in Heaven, and God doesn't want you to be sick here on earth. When you take authority over sickness or disease in your body, you're just taking your place as a child of God with certain rights. You're just exercising your authority and demanding your rights!

Many times, however, Christians will just slip back into the natural, or back into religious thinking which tells them they don't have a say-so about *anything* that happens to them. Rather than *dominating* their circumstances, these Christians are *being dominated* by their circumstances. They have been religiously brainwashed instead of New Testament taught.

We need to *know* the authority God has given us, *believe* in that authority, and *exercise* it. If we don't know the authority God has given us as we should, we need to meditate upon the Scriptures which tell us who we are in Christ, and the authority which God has given us in the Name of Jesus.

The Name of Jesus won't work just because you saw or heard someone else use it. That's where folks miss it sometimes. They say, "Well, Brother Hagin said such-and-such." But they don't study the Word for themselves.

You must be convinced of the Word of God yourself and then act on the Word because you believe it's true. The Name of Jesus will not work for you as it should until you apply yourself to the study of its meaning and its worth.

Using the Name of Jesus To Break the Power of the Devil

When you understand the authority you have in the Name of Jesus, you can also use that Name to break the power of the devil over unsaved people, particularly your unsaved loved ones. I began to study along this line in 1952, and I began to understand the authority we have in Jesus' Name. Now I had been using the Name of Jesus for years, commanding sickness or pain or whatever tried to come against me to leave, and as I used that Name, it left. But I began to see that I could use Jesus' Name to break the power of the devil over my loved ones, and then claim their salvation.

Before I began to see that I could use the Name of Jesus to break the power of the devil over my loved ones and claim their salvation, I spent a lot of time praying that my loved ones would be saved. One day the Holy Spirit showed me something about what I had been doing. The Holy Spirit made it clear to me that if people knew the truth about Heaven and hell and if they understood that Jesus died to save them and give them eternal life, they would not go down the path, so to speak, that they normally would.

Then the Holy Spirit gave me this example: "No one in his right mind would drive his automobile 100 miles per hour past flashing red lights and signs that read, 'WARNING! BRIDGE OUT!' without stopping his automobile in order to avoid destruction." But a person who was *not* in his right mind would! A drunk person, for example, is not in his right mind. A drunk person is not as alert as someone who is sober, and, consequently, he might not heed the red flashing lights and warning signs. The Bible says, "*. . . the god of this world hath blinded the minds of them which believe not, lest the light of the glorious gospel of Christ, who is the image of God, should shine unto them*" (2 Cor. 4:4).

As the Holy Spirit spoke to me about this, I could see in my spirit a multitude of people going down what appeared to be a highway. The multitude came to a place where the highway ended, and they plunged right over what looked like the edge of a cliff and went down into the pit of hell! The god of this world, Satan, had blinded their minds.

The Word says, "*The entrance of thy words giveth light; it giveth understanding unto the simple*" (Psalm 119:130). Many times, if you expose a person to the Word, the Word will give him light, and spiritually he'll be able to see the truth. But sometimes, the power which is controlling an unsaved person needs to be broken, or rendered ineffective before he can see the truth and act on it.

When I understood that I could use the Name of Jesus to break the power of the devil over my unsaved loved ones, I immediately said to myself, "I'll do just that." The meanest relative I had, my brother Dub, came to my mind. I thought *if it works on him, it will work on anyone*!

I had been reading the Bible, meditating, and praying. My Bible was opened to the Book of Philippians, so I stood and read Philippians 2:9.

PHILIPPIANS 2:9
9 Wherefore God also hath highly exalted him [Jesus], **and given him A NAME WHICH IS ABOVE EVERY NAME.**

God highly exalted Jesus the Person and gave Him a Name which is above every name. And the Name and the Person are one. For example, if your name were John Smith, people wouldn't think of you as Harvey Alligator. No. If they know your name, then when they think of *you*, they think of your *name*. Or, if they know your name, when they think of your name, they think of you. The name and the person are one. Thank God, the Lord Jesus Christ and His Name are one!

Now let's go on reading in Philippians chapter 2.

PHILIPPIANS 2:10,11
10 That at THE NAME OF JESUS every knee should bow, of things in heaven, and things in earth, and things under the earth;
11 And that every tongue should confess that Jesus Christ is Lord, to the glory of God the Father.

Verse 10 says, "*That at the name of Jesus every knee should bow, of THINGS in heaven, and THINGS in earth, and THINGS under the earth.*" Other translations say "beings" instead of "things." So we could read verse 10, ". . . every knee should bow, of *beings* in heaven, and *beings* in earth, and *beings* under the earth." Beings in Heaven, in earth, and under the earth include angels and demons. In other words, angels and demons alike are subject to the Name of Jesus. They must surrender to that Name, because the

Name of Jesus is superior to every name that can be named!

As I said earlier, I was standing with my Bible in my hand, opened to that portion of Scripture in the Book of Philippians. So I raised my other hand to Heaven and said, "I take the Name of Jesus and break the power of the devil over my brother Dub, and I claim his deliverance and salvation."

When I took authority over the demons influencing Dub's life and then claimed his salvation, that settled it for me. I didn't even think about it or pray about it anymore. My brother Dub was the "black sheep" of the family. I didn't even know where he was at the time I used the Name of Jesus on his behalf, but to me it was settled, and within three weeks he was saved!

Use the Name of Jesus in Faith

When you get the revelation of the power and authority you have in the Name of Jesus, no one can steal that revelation from you. You must use the Name of Jesus in faith; otherwise, you will be ineffective and you won't get results. Unbelief cries and begs and pleads, but faith speaks and then shouts the victory!

Through faith in the Name of Jesus, you can exercise authority over the power of the enemy in your life, and experience deliverance, healing, and victory! Jesus said, *"If ye shall ask* [demand] *any thing in my name, I will do it"* (John 14:14). I didn't get the revelation of that scripture just by reading it once or twice; I didn't get it by hearing someone else's testimony of how it worked for them. I got the revelation of the power of the Name of Jesus by careful study, meditation, and application of the truth of God's Word.

Someone might say, "Well, I don't know about that. I *tried* using the Name of Jesus once, and it didn't work." Once the reality of the authority that's in the Name of Jesus has dawned on you—once the authority that's in the Name of Jesus has become a reality in your spirit—your days of *trying* will be over, and your days of *doing* will begin!

Every believer should clearly understand the power and authority in the Name of Jesus and the believer's right to use that Name. Meditate upon the scriptures that tell you who you are in Christ and what authority you have as a believer. As you do, those scriptures will become a reality to you. And you will begin to exercise your right to perfect deliverance from the bondage of Satan—for yourself and for your loved ones—in the Name of Jesus!

Questions for Study

1. Who does the Name of Jesus belong to?

   _____
   _____

2. John 14:12-14 does not refer to prayer. What does it refer to?

   _____
   _____

3. What is the Greek definition of the word "ask" in John 14:13 and 14?

   _____
   _____

4. In Acts 3:2-8, when Peter demanded healing for the lame man in the Name of Jesus, he didn't demand anything of God. To whom was he making the demand?

   _____
   _____

5. Why doesn't the Name of Jesus mean as much as it should to some believers?

   _____
   _____

6. What must you have before the Name of Jesus will produce results for you?

   _____
   _____

7. As long as people just try the Name of Jesus as though it's some sort of good luck charm, what will happen for them?

   _____
   _____

8. As the caretaker of your physical body, what right do you have?

   _____
   _____

9. In Romans 12:1, what did Paul say the believer's reasonable service is?

   _____
   _____

10. According to Matthew 6:10, how can you know that God doesn't want you to be sick here on earth?

   _____
   _____

Chapter 13

Prayer for Healing

The Bible teaches that there are several kinds of prayer. However, I will not go into detail on all of them in this chapter. (I do have several books on prayer which discuss them in more detail.) Right now I just want to concentrate on prayer for healing.

Pray to the Father in the Name of Jesus

JOHN 16:23,24
23 And IN THAT DAY ye shall ask me nothing. Verily, verily, I say unto you, Whatsoever ye shall ask the Father IN MY NAME, he will give it you.
24 Hitherto have ye asked nothing IN MY NAME: ask, and ye shall receive, that your joy may be full.

What day was Jesus talking about when He said "*. . . in that day ye shall ask me nothing . . .*" (v. 23)? He was talking about the day that we are living in right now. Praying to the Father in the Name of Jesus belongs to us *now*—in this day.

Jesus said "*. . . in that day ye shall ask me nothing . . .*" just before He went to Calvary. After which a new day dawned, and we came into the *New Covenant.*

Notice John 16:24 says, "*Hitherto have ye asked nothing in my name. . . .*" The word "hitherto" means *until now*. Jesus was really saying, "Until this time you have not prayed in My Name." It wouldn't have done the disciples or anyone else any good to have prayed to the Father in the Name of Jesus while Jesus was here on earth, because, under the *Old Covenant,* they prayed to the God of Abraham, Isaac, and Jacob.

You see, when Jesus was here on earth, He had not yet entered His mediatory (high priestly or intercessory) ministry at the right hand of the Father, so it would not have done any good to have prayed in His Name.

But just before He went away, Jesus changed His disciples' way of praying. During the interim when the Old Covenant was going out and the New Covenant was coming in, Jesus taught the disciples to pray what we call "The Lord's Prayer" (Matt. 6:9). He did not teach *us* to pray this way; He taught His *disciples* to pray this way.

I did not say The Lord's Prayer isn't beautiful. I did not say we cannot learn something from it—because we can learn much from it. But where is the Name of Jesus in it? The disciples didn't pray one thing in the Name of Jesus, did they? They didn't ask for one thing in the Name of Jesus. *This is not the New Testament Church at prayer!* This is not the New Testament norm for prayer.

There's something we need to see here in John chapter 16: Just before Jesus went away, He changed the disciples' way of praying. *Under the New Covenant between God and the Church, we are to come to God by Jesus Christ.* One reason we have missed a great deal is that we have tried to pray as they did back in the days of the Old Covenant.

Notice Jesus said, "*. . . ASK, and ye SHALL RECEIVE, that your joy may be full*" (v. 24). Of course, this includes all prayer, and it includes praying for healing as well. How could your joy be full if you or your loved ones were home sick? That would be impossible, wouldn't it?

You see, every believer has a right to ask God the Father for healing or for any other blessing mentioned in God's Word. And if a believer asks in the Name of Jesus, he has an absolute guarantee that God will grant him the answer to his petition.

If we were getting more answers to prayer, we would have more joy. And if more of our joy were showing, we would get more people saved and healed.

Healing is involved in these verses. We have a right to ask for healing in the Name of Jesus. God does hear and answer prayer.

Agree in Prayer

MATTHEW 18:19,20
19 Again I [Jesus] say unto you, That if two of you shall agree on earth as touching any thing that they shall ask, it shall be done for them of my Father which is in heaven.
20 For where two or three are gathered together in my name, there am I in the midst of them.

Frequently we take verse 20 out of its setting and apply it only to church services—but that really isn't what it's talking about. You see, verses 19 and 20 go together. According to verse 20, wherever two people are, agreeing in prayer, Jesus is there to see that what they agreed on happens. Jesus is not talking about a church meeting here, although He *is* present in church meetings.

Where two people are united and are demanding healing for themselves or their loved ones in Jesus' Name, their prayers are bound to be answered, because God watches over His Word to make it good (Jer. 1:12)!

Matthew 18:19 says "two of you on earth," not "two of you in Heaven." Just two. And the phrase "anything that they shall ask" could include healing, couldn't it?

Well, the "two of you" could be husband and wife. My wife and I have had marvelous answers to prayer by agreeing together. Yet people tell me, "Brother Hagin, we *tried* that, and it didn't work." My wife and I didn't *try* it. We *did* it! Jesus didn't say that two should *try* to agree; He said to *do* it.

Sometimes we get into the natural and think, *Now, if I could get enough people—maybe a thousand—agreeing; maybe ten thousand praying, that would really get results!* That is human reasoning. God said that *two could get the job done.* Two is the most that He ever mentions we need! He didn't say to get the whole church to agree on it. (You couldn't get a whole church to agree on something to save your life!) But if two of you agree, that's all it takes.

Jesus said, ". . . *if two of you shall agree on earth as touching any thing . . . IT SHALL BE . . .*" (v. 19). Jesus didn't say it might be or it's a possibility.

He said, ". . . *IT SHALL BE DONE for them of my Father which is in heaven.*"

Often people ask me to agree with them in prayer for financial, physical, and spiritual needs. I usually join hands with them and pray: "We are joining hands here physically to denote the fact that our spirits are agreeing. We agree that this need *is* met—not that it is going to be, because that is not faith, that would be future tense. That would be hope, not faith. We agree that the need is met, so we are praising God because we have agreed that it shall be done. By faith it is done right now, and we count it as done."

After praying like this I ask the person, "Is it done?"

Eight times out of ten the person starts bawling, "Brother Hagin, I *hope* it is."

I have to tell them, "It isn't. I'm *believing* and you're *hoping*. There is no agreement here. It didn't work."

There is no use in our going around blaming God and casting bad reflections on the Bible if it didn't work. Friends, if it didn't work, *we* didn't work it, because Jesus Christ cannot lie! We must admit that we didn't do it and then correct ourselves.

Add Praise to Your Prayers and Get Results!

When I tell people they don't have to pray to be healed, they look at me in amazement. Many have failed to receive healing because they have based their faith on prayer instead of on God's Word. They expected prayer to do for them what God's Word will do for them. But prayer is successful only when it is based on the promises in God's Word!

It seems that most of our prayers are prayers of petition—asking God to do something for us. And, of course, it's scriptural for us to pray that way, but we also need to add praise to our prayers, because it's in an atmosphere of praise that God can move more readily in our midst.

A young Pentecostal evangelist found that out when he was dying of tuberculosis back in the early 1930s. He told me his story firsthand.

He had become bedfast and was hemorrhaging from both lungs. He had had to take his family to live on his father-in-law's farm.

One day his father-in-law was out in the fields plowing, and his wife and mother-in-law were behind the house doing the wash. So this young evangelist begged God for enough strength to get out of bed and make it to a clump of trees and bushes a quarter of a mile down the road. He purposed in his heart, *I'm going to pray until I pray through and God heals me, or until they find me dead—one of the two.*

He reached the thicket and fell down exhausted. He couldn't have cried for help if he had wanted to. No one knew where he was.

"They won't find you until the buzzards lead them to you," the devil assured him.

"Well," the evangelist said, "that's all right, devil. That's why I came out here. Just as soon as I can regain a little strength, I'm going to pray until I'm healed or die at this spot."

The young man said, "As I was lying there, trying to muster enough strength to start praying, I got to thinking about it: Everywhere I had been, I had turned in prayer requests for my healing. *Hundreds* of people had prayed. *Thousands* of people had prayed. Every healing evangelist in America had laid hands on me. *Everybody* had prayed.

"If you put all those prayers together, it would add up to hundreds of hours of prayer. Many great men of faith had laid hands on me—and God uses healing evangelists. I finally decided, 'I'm not going to pray at all. There is no use in my praying. I see where I've missed it. I shouldn't even have turned in all those prayer requests. I've been trying to get a bunch of people to pray for me. I've been trying to get God to give me what He said is already mine!'

"'The Bible says I'm healed. So, Lord, I'm going to lie here flat on my back and praise You. I'm going to praise You until my healing is manifested.'"

That young evangelist told me, "I just started whispering, 'Praise the Lord. Glory to God. Hallelujah. Thank You, Jesus.' After about ten minutes of whispering, I got enough strength to lift my arms up by propping my elbows on the ground. And I praised God for another ten minutes or so. Then I got enough strength to lift my hands, and my voice got louder. At the end of two hours, I was on my feet hollering, 'Praise God,' so loudly that someone heard me several miles away!"

You see, when he began to agree with what the Word of God says and acted on God's Word, he got results!

The Prayer of Faith

First-century believers did not have a complete New Testament. They had some letters that could be passed around from church to church, but they did not have an entire Bible to study as we do.

They did not know that Peter had written by the Spirit of God "*. . . by whose stripes ye WERE HEALED*" (1 Peter 2:24). But we know that. If they could walk in divine health, how much more should we in this generation, with all the knowledge we have, walk in divine health?

The following passage of Scripture reveals that there are many elements to the prayer of faith.

JAMES 5:14,15
14 Is any sick among you? let him call for the elders of the church; and let them pray over him, anointing him with oil in the name of the Lord:
15 And THE PRAYER OF FAITH SHALL SAVE THE SICK, AND THE LORD SHALL RAISE HIM UP; and if he have committed sins, they shall be forgiven him.

There really ought not be any sick among us—but James asked, "Is there anyone sick among you?" James was clearly talking to the Church here, because he said "*. . . let him call for the elders of the church . . .*" (v. 14). If you can't pray for your own healing, God has made provision for you where you can find help. And, thank God, even if people have missed it and have sinned, there is help for them. Notice in verse 15, James says, "If he has committed sins, they shall be forgiven him."

James 5:16 clearly shows us that healing can be obtained through prayer.

JAMES 5:16
16 Confess your faults one to another, and PRAY ONE FOR ANOTHER, THAT YE MAY BE HEALED. The effectual fervent prayer of a righteous man availeth much.

James 5:16 is talking about believers praying for one another that they might be healed. The thought I want to impress upon you is the last part of this verse: "The effectual fervent prayer of a righteous man availeth much." This is just another way of saying that prayer works!

Who Is Righteous?

But here is where many people run into difficulty with this verse. They say, "Well, if I were *righteous*, I could get my prayers heard and answered." That's the lie the devil used on me.

As I've stately previously, I was sickly until I was seventeen years old. I didn't grow up normally because for the first sixteen years of my life, I couldn't run and play like other children. I played very limitedly because I had a deformed heart and an incurable blood disease. I never had a normal childhood, and about four months before my sixteenth birthday, I became totally bedfast. Several doctors had been called in on my case. And one of the best surgeons in the world said that no one in my condition in the history of medical science had ever lived past the age of sixteen.

I had gotten born again, and I knew that the Holy Spirit lived inside me. But I didn't know at first that I was supposed *to listen* to Him or that He would guide me to act on God's Word. I just knew in my spirit that I didn't have to die at such an early age.

During the time I was bedfast, the Holy Spirit kept trying to tell me I could be healed. Finally one day, I heard something on the inside of me— that still, small voice—say, "You don't have to die at this early age. You can be healed." Then that same inward voice told me that there was help for me in the Word of God.

So I began to diligently study the Bible day and night. I had read the Bible as a young Baptist boy, but I didn't know much about acting on the Word. The doctors had said that I might not live very long so I ran the references on faith, prayer, and healing. Finally, I got over to the Book of James. When I read *"Is any sick among you? let him call for the elders of the church; and let them pray over him, anointing him with oil in the name of the Lord: And the prayer of faith shall save the sick, and the Lord shall raise him up . . ."* (vv. 14,15), I was heartbroken.

I began to cry. I told the Lord, "If I have to do that, I can never be healed; because I don't know anyone—no preacher, minister, deacon, Sunday school superintendent or teacher—who believes in or practices anointing with oil and praying for healing." Then the Spirit of God spoke to my spirit these words: "Did you notice that verse says *the prayer of faith* will save the sick?" I said, "No. I didn't notice that." I read it again, and sure enough that's what it said. That still, small voice said, "You can pray the prayer of faith as well as anyone can." At that moment, I started to believe I could pray the prayer of faith for myself and be healed.

Then I heard another voice say, "Did you notice what the next verse says?" So I read James 5:16: *"Confess your faults one to another, and pray one for another, that ye may be healed. The effectual fervent prayer of a righteous man availeth much."* The voice continued, "You could pray the prayer of faith, *if you were righteous.* But you're not righteous."

I didn't realize that was the voice of the devil, so I more or less accepted what he said. I sided right in with him and said, "You're right. I sure am not righteous." The devil brought to my remembrance an incident when I was irritable and knocked my tray off the bed. There was food everywhere. He said, "That wasn't any way for a righteous person to act, was it?"

I thought being righteous meant you had attained some great degree of spiritual growth, that you always had right conduct. I said to myself, *If I can keep from dying, maybe I can eventually grow to become righteous.*

So there I was. I was sure that because I wasn't righteous, I couldn't get my prayers answered. I laid there bedfast for another three months. I continued to read and study the Word. One day I was reading those same verses in James chapter 5 again, and the Holy Ghost led me to read further. I read verse 17, which says, *"Elias [Elijah] was a man subject to like passions as we are, and he prayed earnestly that it might not rain: and it rained not on the earth by the space of three years and six months."*

I began to analyze that verse for a moment. Verse 16 tells us to confess our faults to one another and pray that we might be healed, because the effectual fervent prayer of a righteous man avails much. Verse 17 points out that Elijah was human and that he was subject to like passions as we are to show us that he had faults and shortcomings just as we do. And James listed Elijah as an example of a righteous man whose prayers were answered! Then I realized that a person who has faults can still be a righteous person. I hadn't seen that three months earlier, and the devil knew it.

Elijah's prayers were answered because he prayed effectually and fervently. That's why many people's prayers go unanswered—people are not effectual or fervent when they pray. The Greek word translated "fervent" really means *white-hot*. When a blacksmith is working with a piece of metal in the fire, the metal gets hot and turns red. After a while, the metal becomes so hot that it turns white. So it's the white-hot prayer of a righteous man that avails much!

We Are Righteous in Christ!

My definition of righteousness was all wrong. So I found out what the Bible had to say on the subject.

2 CORINTHIANS 5:17,21
17 Therefore if any man be in Christ, he is a new creature: old things are passed away; behold, all things are become new. . . .
21 For he hath made him to be sin for us, who knew no sin; that we might be made the righteousness of God in him.

When I read those verses this time, I realized that the blood of Jesus had washed my sins away, cleansed me, and made me a new creature. It didn't make me an unrighteous new creature. I became the righteousness of God in Christ! You see, we can't make ourselves right with God. Only the blood of Jesus can make us right with God. We simply accept His righteousness.

But the devil didn't give up so easy. He knew that I didn't know as much about righteousness as I should. The devil told me, "You're right about that. Jesus made you a new creature; and He didn't make you an unrighteous new creature. But after you were made a new man in Christ, you lost your temper and knocked the tray off the bed. Is that any way for a righteous man to act?"

Well, the devil had me under condemnation again. I thought my prayer wouldn't work, so I didn't even try to pray. But, thank God for the Holy Ghost! He will always lead you back to the Word, because that's where the answer is. The Holy Ghost led me to First John 1:9, which says, *"If we confess our sins, he is faithful and just to forgive us our sins, and to cleanse us from all unrighteousness."* John wrote this to Christians, not sinners.

When I read that verse, I started hollering, "Mr. Devil, I've got you now! You already admitted that when I was born again, I became a new creature in Christ; and He didn't make me an unrighteous new creature. But you told me that when I did wrong and missed it, I lost my righteousness. But the Bible says that if I confess my sins to God, He is faithful and just to forgive my sins and cleanse me from all unrighteousness.

"If God only forgave my sins, I'd still be in a dilemma, because I would still be in a state of unrighteousness. My prayers wouldn't work, because I'd be under condemnation. But God forgives me *and* cleanses me from all unrighteousness! And if I'm cleansed from all unrighteousness, that means I'm righteous again!" And since the prayer of a righteous man avails much, I prayed the prayer of faith for myself, and I was healed!

Questions for Study

1. When is prayer successful?

   _____

   _____

2. According to John 16:23, what *day* does praying to the Father in the Name of Jesus belong to?

   _____

   _____

3. Why wouldn't it have done the disciples or anyone else any good to have prayed to the Father in Jesus' Name while Jesus was here on earth?

   _____

   _____

4. How did Jesus change the disciples' way of praying in John 16:23 and 24?

   _____

   _____

5. Why isn't The Lord's Prayer for the New Testament Church?

   _____

   _____

6. Under the New Covenant between God and the Church, how are we to come to God?

   _____

   _____

7. According to Matthew 18:19 and 20, what happens when two or more believers agree in prayer?

   _____

   _____

8. Why is it unnecessary to try to get the whole church to agree in prayer?

   _____

   _____

9. When it comes to prayer, what is the difference between believing and hoping?

   _____

   _____

10. Why do many people fail to receive healing even after they have prayed?

    _____

    _____

Chapter 14

The Laying On of Hands—Part 1

A Pentecostal minister once told me: "Twenty-five years ago, God spoke to me about a ministry of laying on of hands, but I backed off from it. Even though God used me in it, some of the brethren didn't understand it, and I didn't want to make a doctrine out of it."

"You didn't have to," I said. "Jesus made a doctrine out of it."

The laying on of hands is a fundamental principle of the doctrine of Christ.

HEBREWS 6:1,2
1 Therefore leaving THE PRINCIPLES OF THE DOCTRINE OF CHRIST, let us go on unto perfection; not laying again the foundation of repentance from dead works, and of faith toward God,
2 Of THE DOCTRINE of baptisms, and OF LAYING ON OF HANDS, and of resurrection of the dead, and of eternal judgment.

"Laying on of hands" is one of the fundamental principles of the doctrine of the Lord Jesus Christ listed in Hebrews 6:1 and 2. Those principles are:

1. *Repentance*—This leads to the New Birth experience.

2. *Faith Toward God*—The Bible says we can't be saved without faith: "*. . . by grace are ye saved through faith; and that not of yourselves: it is the gift of God: Not of works, lest any man should boast*" (Eph. 2:8,9).

3. *Doctrine of Baptisms*—Notice this is in the plural. There are three baptisms spoken of in the New Testament. First, there is the New Birth. When a person is born again, he is baptized by the Holy Spirit into the Body of Christ. Second, there is water baptism, which is an outward sign of an inward grace. Third, there is the baptism in the Holy Spirit with the Bible evidence of speaking in other tongues.

4. *Laying on of Hands*—We will examine this doctrine later.

5. *Resurrection of the Dead*—Notice Hebrews 6:2 does not say "the" resurrection. It says,

"*. . . and of resurrection of the dead. . . .*" Had it said "the resurrection," there would be just one resurrection; but there is more than one resurrection, so it says "resurrection of the dead."

This includes the first resurrection, the second resurrection, and all other resurrections. It includes the fact that the dead in Christ shall be raised first; then we who are alive and remain at the coming of Christ will be caught up too (this is the rapture of the saints).

6. *Eternal Judgment*—Again, it is not "the" doctrine of "the" eternal judgment; it is simply "doctrine of eternal judgment." This is because there is more than one judgment, and all are involved in this doctrine.

These six fundamental principles are the foundation upon which the Church is built. Therefore, not one of them should be treated lightly or cast aside as something unimportant to the Body of Christ.

If I were to say, "I don't much believe in the New Birth, water baptism, or the baptism in the Holy Spirit," you'd be ready to quit me right now and run me out, and I wouldn't blame you. And you would be certain something was wrong with me if I were to say, "I don't think the dead will ever be resurrected." Or "I don't go along with this judgment business. I don't think there's going to be any judgment."

You would say, "There's something wrong with that fellow. He's not solid. He doesn't believe the fundamental principles of the doctrine of Christ."

Well, no matter what else we believe, we must believe the fundamentals. (I can fellowship with anyone who believes the fundamentals.) And if *one* of the fundamental principles is right, they are *all* right. You can't leave any one of them out.

The Doctrine of Laying On of Hands

The Bible has a great deal to say about the doctrine of laying on of hands. That's why it's surprising to me that some Christians see no significance at all in this scriptural ordinance and doctrine. We hear lots of sermons on repentance, and we hear much preaching on faith. Thank God for it! But we rarely hear any teaching on the laying on of hands. The lack of teaching on the subject has given many believers the wrong impression that it's unimportant and of no particular value to us. But if it's a fundamental principle of the doctrine of Christ, it is valuable!

I suppose the lack of teaching on the subject is the reason why so many Christians regard the laying on of hands with something like astonishment. Others regard it with fear. But the laying on of hands is one of the half dozen fundamental principles of the doctrine of the Lord Jesus Christ!

I have even heard Full Gospel ministers say, "I don't much go along with the laying on of hands." To deny one of the fundamental principles of the doctrine of Jesus Christ is a serious matter.

Scriptural Purposes for the Laying On of Hands

Actually, the laying on of hands is a theme that runs through the entire Bible. There are several scriptural purposes for employing the laying on of hands. Let's examine some examples from both the Old and New Testaments.

Old Testament Examples

In the Old Testament, we see that the laying on of hands was used for several different purposes.

The Book of Genesis reveals that the laying on of hands was used *to impart blessings.* Genesis 48:14 says, *"And Israel [Jacob] stretched out his right hand, and laid it upon Ephraim's head, who was the younger, and his left hand upon Manasseh's head, guiding his hands wittingly; for Manasseh was the firstborn."* Israel laid his hands on his grandsons and spoke words of blessing over them.

In Exodus 29, we also see that God instructed the Levites to use the laying on of hands *during the worship service.*

EXODUS 29:10,15,19
10 And thou [Moses] shalt cause a bullock to be brought before the tabernacle of the congregation: and Aaron and his sons shall PUT THEIR HANDS UPON the head of the bullock....
15 Thou shalt also take one ram; and Aaron and his sons shall put their hands upon the head of the ram....
19 And thou shalt take the other ram; and Aaron and his sons shall put their hands upon the head of the ram.

We read here that the *imperfections* of the worshippers were transferred by faith to the sacrifice. The sacrifice was a type of Christ. The *perfections* of the sacrifice were received by faith by the man who laid hands on the sacrifice. It was God's power that effected the two-way transmission.

The Bible reveals that another purpose for which the laying on of hands was used was *to equip men to serve God.* The following passage of Scripture tells us that when the time had come for Moses to leave this earth, God directed Moses to lay his hands upon Joshua, Israel's next leader, to impart a measure of his honor to him.

NUMBERS 27:18-23
18 And the Lord said unto Moses, Take thee Joshua the son of Nun, a man in whom is the spirit, and LAY THINE HAND UPON HIM;
19 And set him before Eleazar the priest, and before all the congregation; and give him a charge in their sight.
20 And THOU SHALT PUT SOME OF THINE HONOUR UPON HIM, that all the congregation of the children of Israel may be obedient.
21 And he shall stand before Eleazar the priest, who shall ask counsel for him after the judgment of Urim before the Lord: at his word shall they go out, and at his word they shall come in, both he, and all the children of Israel with him, even all the congregation.
22 And Moses did as the Lord commanded him: and he took Joshua, and set him before Eleazar the priest, and before all the congregation:
23 And he laid his hands upon him, and gave him a charge, as the Lord commanded by the hand of Moses.

Later in the Book of Deuteronomy, we read that Joshua had the same spirit of wisdom that Moses had because Moses had laid his hands upon him. This implies that what Moses had was transferred to Joshua by the laying on of hands.

DEUTERONOMY 34:9
9 And Joshua the son of Nun was full of the spirit of wisdom; FOR MOSES HAD LAID HIS HANDS UPON HIM: and the children of Israel hearkened unto him, and did as the Lord commanded Moses.

Today through the ordinance of the laying on of hands, God's power is transmitted by faith through the minister to the seeker. Something mighty occurs when men of faith lay hands in the Name of the Lord upon those who, by faith, receive the impartation.

New Testament Examples

In the New Testament, we see some distinct purposes for which the laying on of hands was used. The number one reason the laying on of hands was used in the New Testament was to minister *healing*. There are more scripture references concerning healing in connection with the laying on of hands than concerning anything else. But we'll skip over healing right now and look at the other purposes for the laying on of hands.

Another use of the laying on of hands in the New Testament was for *helping believers receive the Holy Spirit*. In Acts 8:17, when Peter and John laid their hands on Philip's Samaritan converts, they received the Holy Spirit.

ACTS 8:14-17
14 Now when the apostles which were at Jerusalem heard that Samaria had received the word of God, they sent unto them Peter and John:
15 Who, when they were come down, prayed for them, that they might receive the Holy Ghost:
16 (For as yet he was fallen upon none of them: only they were baptized in the name of the Lord Jesus.)
17 THEN LAID THEY THEIR HANDS ON THEM, AND THEY RECEIVED THE HOLY GHOST.

Then in Acts 19:6, Paul laid hands on the disciples at Ephesus, and *". . . they spake with tongues, and prophesied."*

ACTS 19:1-6
1 And it came to pass, that, while Apollos was at Corinth, Paul having passed through the upper coasts came to Ephesus: and finding certain disciples,
2 He said unto them, Have ye received the Holy Ghost since ye believed? And they said unto him, We have not so much as heard whether there be any Holy Ghost.
3 And he said unto them, Unto what then were ye baptized? And they said, Unto John's baptism.
4 Then said Paul, John verily baptized with the baptism of repentance, saying unto the people, that they should believe on him which should come after him, that is, on Christ Jesus.
5 When they heard this, they were baptized in the name of the Lord Jesus.
6 And WHEN PAUL HAD LAID HIS HANDS UPON THEM, THE HOLY GHOST CAME ON THEM; and they spake with tongues, and prophesied.

In nearly every instance in the Book of Acts where people were *filled with the Holy Spirit*, they received *by the laying on of hands*. (Exceptions were the spontaneous outpourings of the Spirit in Acts 2 and Acts 10.) Of course people can be filled with the Spirit in other ways, but the laying on of hands is one scriptural method.

Another common New Testament practice was laying hands on those who were being *ordained and separated unto the ministry*.

ACTS 13:2,3
2 As they ministered to the Lord, and fasted, the Holy Ghost said, Separate me Barnabas and Saul for the work whereunto I have called them.
3 And when they had fasted and prayed, and laid their hands on them, they sent them away.

The laying on of hands was also used in *imparting spiritual gifts*. Now when I say "spiritual gifts," I'm not talking about what we call the gifts of the Spirit. What I'm talking about is similar to what took place in Exodus chapter 29, when Moses imparted some of his honor and wisdom to Joshua. In the New Testament example of this, Paul told Timothy, *"Neglect not the gift that is in thee, which was given thee by prophecy, with the laying on of the hands of the presbytery"* (1 Tim. 4:14). Later Paul exhorted Timothy, *". . . I put thee in remembrance that thou stir up the gift of God, which is in thee by the putting on of my hands"* (2 Tim. 1:6). Timothy had received special giftings to minister through the laying on of hands.

The doctrine of laying on of hands does not end with the ordination of ministers, however, as so many denominations believe. That is only one facet of laying on of hands.

There is also scriptural precedent for laying hands on those being *installed in certain church offices*. In Acts chapter 6, seven men were selected to wait on tables, freeing the apostles to give themselves continually to prayer and the ministry of the Word. The apostles laid their hands on the seven, who were called deacons—"helpers" in the Greek.

So you see, the laying on of hands has several distinct purposes.

Laying Empty Hands on Empty Heads

I realize that there is an unprofitable kind of laying on of hands. There are extremes of it in the church world.

One extreme is a mere ritual. There are churches that have a ritual of laying hands on people to confirm them. According to some church creeds, one receives the Holy Spirit at this time. But this is a mere ritual and formality, and nothing happens.

On the other hand, there have been extremes even in Full Gospel circles. People have had hands laid on them for nearly everything you could mention—and some you couldn't.

For example, a woman told me that she went to a meeting where hands were laid on her. She was prophesied over, and she supposedly was given "the gift of casting out permanent waves." I told her if she could have gotten the gift of putting them in, she would have had something!

Once a man came up to me after a service several years ago and asked, "Brother Hagin, could you help me?"

I said, "I'll be glad to if I can."

He told me he had been in a meeting where someone laid hands on him and gave him the gifts of healing, the gift of the word of knowledge, and two or three other spiritual gifts. He said, "I can see that these things are manifested in your ministry. Maybe you could tell me how to operate them. I know I've got them, because that fellow said I did."

I asked, "How long has it been since hands were laid on you?"

"Well," he said, "over six months ago."

I said, "Has there ever been any kind of manifestation?"

"Not that I know of," he replied.

I said, "I'd forget it if I were you. You don't have anything. If it's there, it would rise to the surface."

Then in another place I preached, a woman sat on the second pew, right in front of the pulpit, and rocked just like she was in a rocking chair throughout my sermon. I thought the poor dear was afflicted with some kind of serious physical ailment.

Afterwards I asked the pastor, "What's wrong with that woman? People were looking at her. She was distracting from the message."

"Oh," the pastor said, "Brother Hagin, that's a sad case. There's nothing wrong with her physically. She's not a member here, but she does come to church some. I've been intending to talk to her about it, but I just haven't had time. She attended a meeting somewhere, and someone laid hands on her and gave her 'the gift of rocking.'"

Several nights later that woman came up to me after the service accompanied by a woman who had told her there is nothing in the Bible about "the gift of rocking."

She said, "Brother Hagin, explain my gift to this woman."

Well, I thought that would be a good opportunity for the pastor to talk to her! I said, "I'm on my way out of the building. You go to the pastor of this church. He's a man of God and knows the Bible quite well. He'll be glad to help you."

Afterwards, the pastor said, "You dog!"

I said, "Well, you *said* you wanted to talk to her, so I arranged it. Were you able to help her?"

He said, "Certainly not. No one could help her."

I asked, "Well, what did she tell you? What is the purpose of this so-called gift?"

The pastor answered, "She said that God had given it to her so the pastor or the guest speaker could tell when things were in the Spirit. If she is rocking when we're singing, testifying, or preaching, then everything is in the Spirit."

I know this sounds ridiculous, but it is true. I'm not making it up.

I call all these examples *laying empty hands on empty heads.*

I am not going to be frightened out of a New Testament practice, however, because of fanaticism, nor am I going to be frozen out because of formality. The real is not done away with because of excesses. I'm going to practice the New Testament doctrine of laying on of hands and it's going to produce New Testament results!

88

Questions for Study

1. Name the six fundamental principles of the doctrine of Christ.

2. What are the three different baptisms spoken of in the New Testament?

3. Name two reasons why the laying on of hands was practiced in the Old Testament.

4. What was the animal sacrifice a type of?

5. In Deuteronomy 34:9, when Moses laid hands on Joshua, what did Joshua receive?

6. How is God's power transmitted from the minister to the seeker today?

7. What is the most common practice of laying on of hands in churches?

8. What was the purpose of laying on of hands in Acts chapter 6?

9. In nearly every instance in the Book of Acts when people were filled with the Holy Spirit, they received by the laying on of hands. List the two exceptions in the Book of Acts when believers were filled with the Holy Spirit through spontaneous outpourings of the Spirit.

10. What are the two extremes of the unprofitable kind of laying on of hands in the church world?

Chapter 15

The Laying On of Hands—Part 2

In Chapter 14, we discussed the fact that there are several distinct purposes for which the laying on of hands was used in the New Testament. The number one reason was *healing*. There are more scripture references concerning healing in connection with the laying on of hands than concerning anything else.

As I said in the previous chapter, we can't stop practicing the New Testament doctrine of laying on of hands just because some people fall into a ditch on one side or the other. We need to study the New Testament carefully to see how Jesus and the apostles practiced this doctrine.

Every Christian should practice the doctrine of laying on of hands on the sick, because Jesus said we should (Mark 16:18)!

The Example of Jesus and the Apostles

Jesus Christ Himself freely employed laying on of hands in healing people. In Mark 6, we see Jesus in His hometown of Nazareth:

MARK 6:5
5 And he could there do no mighty work, save that HE LAID HIS HANDS UPON A FEW SICK FOLK, AND HEALED THEM.

Notice this text is speaking of the Lord Jesus Christ Himself—the Son of God. It doesn't say He *wouldn't* do mighty works in Nazareth; it says He *couldn't*. It seems, therefore, that the laying on of hands will work when nothing else will! The few who were healed that day were healed by the laying on of Jesus' hands.

There are several accounts of Jesus' laying hands on people in the New Testament. Matthew 8:15 says that when Jesus entered Peter's house, He found Peter's mother-in-law sick with a fever. *"And he touched her hand, and the fever left her: and she arose, and ministered unto them."* Let's look at a few more examples.

MARK 8:22-25
22 And he [Jesus] cometh to Bethsaida; and they bring a blind man unto him, AND BESOUGHT HIM TO TOUCH HIM.
23 And he took the blind man by the hand, and led him out of the town; and when he had spit on his eyes, AND PUT HIS HANDS UPON HIM, he asked him if he saw ought.
24 And he looked up, and said, I see men as trees, walking.
25 After that HE PUT HIS HANDS AGAIN UPON HIS EYES, and made him look up: and he was restored, and saw every man clearly.

Praise God, the blind man was healed by the laying on of Jesus' hands. Some will say, "Jesus prayed for that blind man twice." I do not know that He *prayed* for him at all, for the Bible does not say He prayed. The Bible says *He laid hands on him twice*! Therefore, it is scripturally correct to lay your hands a second time on a sick person, if necessary. It is good to know what Jesus did in certain circumstances. Then we will know what to do.

MARK 7:32,33,35
32 And they bring unto him [Jesus] one that was deaf, and had an impediment in his speech; and they beseech him to PUT HIS HAND UPON HIM.
33 And he took him aside from the multitude, and put his fingers into his ears, and he spit, and touched his tongue. . . .
35 And straightway his ears were opened, and the string of his tongue was loosed, and he spake plain.

In the case of the deaf man, the scriptures do not say that the people asked Jesus to heal the man, although it is implied. It says they asked Him to put His hands on him.

In these two cases, notice that groups of people brought the blind man and the deaf man to Jesus. These people, as well as the sick themselves, believed in the laying on of hands. The multitudes expected healing through the laying on of hands—and they got the desired results!

I've had people tell me, "I had hands laid on me for healing, and I didn't recover."

I always ask them, "Well, did you expect to recover?" They usually answer, "No. I just thought I'd try it out and see if anything would happen."

People who are just "trying it out" are not going to get healed, because they're not in faith.

You see, if you don't expect to be healed or delivered through the laying on of hands, then having hands laid upon you will be in vain. If you want the laying on of hands to work for you, you've got to believe in it. Without faith, the laying on of hands is a mere ritual, and nothing happens.

Jairus' Daughter

Mark chapter 5 tells us that Jairus, a ruler of the synagogue in Galilee, also believed in the laying on of hands.

MARK 5:22,23
22 And, behold, there cometh one of the rulers of the synagogue, Jairus by name; and when he saw him [Jesus], he fell at his feet,
23 And besought him greatly, saying, My little daughter lieth at the point of death: I pray thee, come and LAY THY HANDS ON HER, that she may be healed; and she shall live.

You see, Jairus believed in the laying on of hands. He didn't say, "Come and *pray* for her." He didn't even say, "Come and *heal* her." He said, "*. . . come and lay thy hands on her, that she may be healed . . .*" (v. 23). Jairus believed his daughter would be healed when hands were laid on her, and he made a confession of his faith.

We know from Scripture that Jesus was on his way to Jairus' house when some people came from Jairus' house and said, "*. . . Thy daughter is dead: why troublest thou the Master any further? As soon as Jesus heard the word that was spoken, he saith unto the ruler of the synagogue, Be not afraid, only believe*" (vv. 35,36). The child had died before Jesus reached Jairus' house, but Jesus still went to the house. Verse 41 says Jesus "*. . . took the damsel by the hand. . . .*" In other words, Jesus touched her. He took her by the hand, and she was raised from the dead healed (v. 42)!

Some might try to argue that since this healing took place during Jesus' earthly ministry, it has no application for us today. Yes, Jesus laid hands on sick people, but He exhorted all believers to lay hands on the sick too! In Mark 16:18 Jesus said, "*. . . they [believers] shall lay hands on the sick, and they shall recover.*"

Who shall lay hands on the sick? It's not just the preachers or those called to the ministry. The answer is in Mark 16:15-18, where Jesus declared The Great Commission:

MARK 16:15-18
15 And he said unto them, Go YE into all the world, and preach the gospel to every creature.
16 He that believeth and is baptized shall be saved; but he that believeth not shall be damned.
17 And these signs shall follow THEM THAT BELIEVE; In my name shall they cast out devils; they shall speak with new tongues;
18 They shall take up serpents; and if they drink any deadly thing, it shall not hurt them; THEY SHALL LAY HANDS ON THE SICK, AND THEY SHALL RECOVER.

Notice that verse 18 says that the sick *shall* recover. Yet some folks think it says, "Lay hands on the sick, and they'll get worse," or "Lay hands on the sick, and if it's the will of God, they'll recover. If not, they'll die." No! Let's be as definite as Scripture is about it. Let's just say what the Bible says: "Believers shall lay hands on the sick, and they shall recover!"

People still preach repentance and water baptism. No one objects to that. Well, why not preach *all* of The Great Commission? Why stop with just part of it? Why not preach the laying on of hands? Laying on of hands is part of The Great Commission too!

The disciples obviously took Jesus seriously. Acts 5:12 says, "*And by the hands of the apostles were many signs and wonders wrought among the people. . . .*"

The Apostle Paul and the Laying On of Hands

In Acts 28:8 and 9 we find the Apostle Paul shipwrecked on an island. The father of the ruler of the island was ill, so Paul went to his house

"*. . . and prayed, and laid his hands on him, and healed him*" (v. 8). The man was healed by the laying on of hands. Then the Bible tells us that the islanders brought their sick to Paul, and he ministered to them. Obviously, Paul ministered by the laying on of hands.

ACTS 19:11,12
11 And God wrought special miracles BY THE HANDS OF PAUL:
12 So that from his body were brought unto the sick handkerchiefs or aprons, and the diseases departed from them, and the evil spirits went out of them.

Not only were the sick healed, but the demon-oppressed were delivered as cloths Paul had laid his hands on were laid upon their bodies. These cloths were anointed with the same *power* Paul was anointed with. When we talk about anointed cloths, however, we do not mean cloths anointed with oil.

God wrought special miracles by the hands of Paul (v. 11). Paul laid his hands upon the cloths. God uses men's hands. He works through men's hands.

Some will say, "The apostles could do that, but it is not for us today." It seems to me that intelligent people should have caught on to that worn-out lie by now. Jesus didn't say these signs would follow just the apostles. He said these signs would follow those who believe!

The Whole Doctrine of Christ

When I found out the truth about divine healing through the laying on of hands, I knew that I didn't have to run around looking for someone special to lay hands on me. It doesn't make me any difference who lays hands on me for healing, because I know what the Bible says. I know that if anyone who believes in healing through the laying on of hands lays hands on me, I'll be healed! You see, my faith is not in the person praying for me; my faith is in the Word of God!

To say that any believer cannot lay hands on the sick today is to say that one of the other fundamental principles of the doctrine of Christ has been done away with. And if laying on of hands for healing has been done away with, no one would have a right to believe in the doctrine of

repentance or any of the fundamental principles of the doctrine of Christ.

For example, the doctrine of baptisms includes water baptism. If you attended a church service where people were baptized in water upon the profession of their faith, you would probably never doubt the efficacy of that ceremony because you read about this ordinance in the Word (Heb. 6:1,2). Well, the doctrine of laying on of hands is just as holy and sacred as the other fundamental principles of the doctrine of Christ!

I'm not going to take anything away from the doctrine of Christ. I believe all of it. I am a follower of Christ. I am a stickler for the doctrine of Christ. And one of the doctrines of Christ is laying on of hands.

'These Signs Shall Follow'

As I said before, Jesus did not say these signs shall follow just the apostles, the preachers, or the teachers. He said, "*. . . these signs shall follow them that believe . . .*" (Mark 16:17).

When I was a Baptist boy, I knew nothing about divine healing, for I had never heard it preached. I just knew what Mark 11:22-24 says about faith and prayer.

My body was almost totally paralyzed. I had a serious organic heart condition and an incurable blood disease. The doctors said I had to die, but I prayed the prayer of faith for myself and was healed. I came off that deathbed as a Baptist boy who preached faith and healing. I didn't know anyone else who believed in divine healing, but it never bothered me.

I stood on the Word of God and said, "Come hell or high water, I'm standing on it. No one is going to move me off of it!"

One day back in 1935, a Presbyterian woman told me her Pentecostal mother-in-law was coming for a visit. "You'll be interested in meeting Grandma," she said, "because she believes like you do. She believes in divine healing."

She told me how her 82-year-old mother-in-law got people healed while visiting them in their homes and laying hands on them. What a healing ministry this elderly Pentecostal woman had!

I never was so thrilled in my life to finally meet someone who had enough sense to believe the Bible! I knew she was arriving on a certain day, so I went over late that afternoon. After I was introduced, I said to this dear old lady, "Grandma, tell me your story."

"Well," she said, "we came out here to Texas many, many years ago (about 1865). My dad settled on some land that was forty miles from the nearest school, so I didn't go to school. I didn't get any education.

"I grew up, married a neighbor boy whose folks also owned a lot of land, and we had our family. I still didn't know how to read or write, but I sent our children to school. They were all grown when some people came along and started what they called a brush arbor meeting. They put up some posts, strung some wires from post to post, and put brush on top of it. I got saved and baptized with the Holy Ghost during that meeting.

"When I got baptized with the Holy Ghost and spoke with other tongues, God taught me to read the Bible. I can read the Bible and never make a mistake, but it's all I can read. I can't read anything else.

"Then we moved to town. My husband and the boys would go out to work the farm in the daytime, and I'd be left alone. I got to asking the Lord, 'Lord, is there something I can do?' I couldn't sing in the church, because I didn't have a voice for music. I couldn't teach a Sunday school class because they used a quarterly, and I couldn't read the quarterly.

"One day I was at home praying and reading the Book of Mark in the Bible, and I read, '. . . *these signs shall follow them that believe. . . . they shall lay hands on the sick, and they shall recover.*' And I thought, *It doesn't take any education to lay hands on folks.*

"The Bible says believers will lay hands on the sick. So I just went through the neighborhood and inquired about any sick folk I could find. I would spend from nine in the morning until three in the afternoon every day visiting sick people and reading the Bible to them on the subject of healing. Usually they had never heard about it.

"After reading to them about three days, I would ask, 'Now would you like for me to lay hands on you?' You know, practically everybody I laid hands on got healed! The amazing thing about it is that most of the people I was laying hands on were bedfast and given up to die by the doctors."

Here was an elderly uneducated woman who wasn't a minister of the Gospel—she had never even taught a Sunday school class—but she was laying hands on the sick, and they were recovering!

Laying on of hands belongs to all of us. Remember now, this dear old lady was not a preacher; but she was a believer. God is the same God now as He was then. He hasn't changed. And when He finds someone He can work with, God and man can do it again.

Who can lay hands on the sick? *Believers* can!

Methods

Laying on of hands can be done in two ways:

First, any believer can lay hands upon a fellow believer as a point of contact to release faith and expect that person to be healed.

There are some people—friends and neighbors, for example—you can pray for whom no one else could. It also is scriptural for husbands and wives to lay hands on each other and for parents to lay hands on their children when they are sick and expect them to be healed in the Name of Jesus.

Second, there is such a thing as a *ministry of laying on of hands*—a special anointing. As God wills, a person can be supernaturally anointed with healing power like Jesus or Paul was anointed.

When the person who has a ministry of laying on of hands lays hands on the sick in obedience to the spiritual Law of Contact and Transmission, his hands transmit God's healing power into the body of the sick person, effecting a healing and a cure. I explain this method further in another chapter.

Questions for Study

1. Why should every Christian practice the doctrine of laying on of hands on the sick?

   _____

   _____

2. Mark 6:5 doesn't say that Jesus wouldn't do mighty works in Nazareth; it says He couldn't. What does this seem to say about the laying on of hands?

   _____

   _____

3. What Bible proof do we have that it is scripturally correct to lay your hands a second time on a sick person, if necessary?

   _____

   _____

4. When the people brought the deaf man to Jesus in Mark chapter 7, what did they ask for?

   _____

   _____

5. If you want the laying on of hands to work for you, what do you have to do?

   _____

   _____

6. Without faith, what is the laying on of hands?

   _____

   _____

7. What does the term "anointed cloths" refer to?

   _____

   _____

8. According to Mark 16:17 and 18, who should lay hands on the sick?

   _____

   _____

9. List the two methods of laying on of hands.

   _____

   _____

10. How does the spiritual law of contact and transmission operate?

   _____

   _____

Chapter 16

Faith and Power—Two Ingredients for Receiving Healing—Part 1

We need to realize that there is no set way by which people may receive healing. In other words, a number of methods for receiving healing are recorded in the Word of God.

One way you can receive healing is by what I call *simple faith*—when you hear the Word of God yourself, believe that what it says is true, and receive your healing by faith in God's Word.

A second way is *to be ministered to with the laying on of hands*—the healing anointing flows through another person to you.

A third way to receive healing is in conjunction with what older Pentecostals often called, *"praying the power down"*—receiving your healing when the supernatural power of God is manifested upon you.

All of these methods are scriptural, all of them require faith, and, thank God, all of them work! In the next two chapters, we are going to discuss these three methods, with our main focus on the two ingredients which are required for each of them to work—*faith and power*.

The Healing Power of God

Concerning the power, Acts 10:38 indicates that the terms "the anointing," "the Holy Ghost," and "power" are virtually synonymous. This means that we are able to use these terms interchangeably when discussing the subject of the healing anointing and the power of God.

A good analogy for understanding the anointing or the power of God was made by the late Rev. John G. Lake when he said, *"Electricity* is God's power in the *natural* realm; *Holy Ghost power* is God's power in the *spirit* realm."

You see, just as electricity is in existence in the natural world, the power of God is in existence in the spirit world. And just as there are laws that govern the operation of electricity in the natural realm, there are also laws that govern the operation of spiritual power. The

problem has been that in times past, we have thought that if the anointing was present, it would automatically manifest itself and just work automatically. That's just not so.

For example, electricity has been in existence in the earth since God created the universe. But did that electricity just automatically light up a house, cook a meal, or warm or cool a house? No, because for many years, man didn't even know electricity existed.

Even after electricity was discovered and man knew it existed, it didn't automatically begin to operate. Man had to come in contact with it somehow to make it work.

Well, if we could just get into our minds the fact that the healing power of God is in existence in the spirit world and that it also has laws that govern its operation, then men and women could learn to tap into that power and be blessed by its benefits.

I've heard people ask, "If the power of God to heal exists, why doesn't it just move on our behalf?"

That's where we've missed it. We've thought, *Well, if it's so, it'll just manifest itself.*

But, no, there's something that has to be done on man's end before there will be a manifestation of the healing power.

In the natural, there came a time when man knew about electricity; it had even been manifested in a measure. But man had to learn more about electricity and the laws that governed it before he could fully enjoy it—before he could gain the greatest benefit from it.

It's the same way with God's power—the anointing. That simply means that as we learn more about the anointing and what the Word of God says about it, we will be able to flow with the anointing, tap into the power, and gain greater benefits from it.

The Switch of Faith

Now that we understand something about the power of God as "heavenly electricity," as it were, let's extend the analogy a step further concerning faith. Another thing about the laws that govern this heavenly substance is this fact: The thing that turns the heavenly power on in the spiritual realm can be compared to an electrical switch on a wall that turns on the earthly power—electricity—in the natural realm.

In the natural, when you turn a light switch on, electricity flows right into the lighting fixtures and lights up the room. When you turn the switch off, the lights go out. So in the spiritual realm, the thing that turns on the heavenly power could be called the *switch of faith*!

Remember Jesus said to the woman with the issue of blood, "*. . . Daughter, THY FAITH hath made thee whole . . .*" (Mark 5:34). Jesus said that her faith had made her whole. In other words, she had turned on the switch of faith for healing and activated the power of God!

When I was a teenager, I was bedfast for sixteen months with an incurable blood disease. Beside my bed was an electrical outlet. Anyone could have plugged a light in there, and it would have lit up the room. The electricity was there, but there was no manifestation of it whatsoever because no one had plugged anything into the outlet.

Well, by the same token, the power of God to heal was present in my room every single day, because God is everywhere present, and whatever power He has is with Him!

But there was no manifestation of it. Why not? Because I didn't plug in to it! I didn't know how!

But, you see, on the eighth day of August, 1934, I learned how. *By faith, I plugged into God's power to heal!* And I began to say, "Now I believe I'm well."

If a man believes he's well, then he'll act like he's well. Even though I was paralyzed, I had regained some use of the upper part of my body, so I pushed my feet off the bed. They fell to the floor like a couple of chunks of wood. I could

look down there and see that they were down there on the floor, but I couldn't *feel* them. I was "dead" from my waist down. Then I managed to get hold of one of the bedposts and scoot my body off the bed. I wrapped my arms around that post, but my knees sagged to the floor.

Out loud, I said, "I want to announce in the Presence of Almighty God, the Lord Jesus Christ, the holy angels, and the devil and all of his cohorts that according to the Word of God, I am healed!"

Now when I said that, I "plugged in." I felt that power strike me in the top of my head and ooze down all over me. It felt like someone was above me pouring a pitcher of warm honey on me. It went down my body and my arms. When it got to my waist and down my legs, it felt like ten thousand pins were sticking in my legs. It felt so bad, I could have cried if it hadn't felt so good at the same time! When you have had no feeling at all, it feels good to feel *anything*!

After that happened, I was standing up straight! Hallelujah! I plugged in to that power. *You can plug in to God's power on your own faith!*

Now you can teach people the Word, and they can believe God's Word and receive healing. I was healed as a young boy by simply believing and acting upon God's Word.

However, not everyone is at the level in his faith where he can just believe God's Word for himself and receive healing through faith in the Word alone. Therefore, we should endeavor to teach and preach all of it—every side of divine healing—and to minister to people on all levels of faith and by all methods of healing.

Faith in the Anointing

Let's look again at the fifth chapter of Mark's Gospel about the healing of the woman with the issue of blood. Matthew, Mark, and Luke all record this same incident, but Mark goes into a little more detail about it and gives us more input than the other two Gospels.

MARK 5:25-34

25 And a certain woman, which had an issue of blood twelve years,

26 And had suffered many things of many physicians, and had spent all that she had, and was nothing bettered, but rather grew worse,

27 When she had heard of Jesus, came in the press behind, and touched his garment.

28 For she said, If I may touch but his clothes, I shall be whole.

29 And straightway the fountain of her blood was dried up; and she felt in her body that she was healed of that plague.

30 And Jesus, IMMEDIATELY knowing in himself that virtue [power] had gone out of him, turned him about in the press, and said, Who touched my clothes?

31 And his disciples said unto him, Thou seest the multitude thronging thee, and sayest thou, Who touched me?

32 And he looked round about to see her that had done this thing.

33 But the woman fearing and trembling, knowing what was done in her, came and fell down before him, and told him all the truth.

34 And he said unto her, Daughter, thy faith hath made thee whole; go in peace, and be whole of thy plague.

I want you to notice that Jesus immediately was aware that the anointing flowed *out from* Him. Also, notice that the woman with the issue of blood *cooperated with the anointing* that flowed from Jesus into her, and she was healed.

The healing anointing flowed out of Jesus' clothes and into the woman with the issue of blood. But Jesus said to her, "*Thy faith* hath made thee whole." It wasn't the healing anointing alone that healed this woman. It was *her faith* in the healing anointing that healed her. Or we could say it like this: It was her faith a*nd* the healing anointing that healed her!

The healing power of God—the anointing—is a tangible substance. It is a heavenly materiality. Believe that, and it can begin to work for you.

Turn on the 'Switch of Faith'!

We know that a person can receive divine healing any number of ways. We've talked about simply receiving healing by faith in the Word without any transfer of power, and we've talked about receiving through the healing anointing.

But notice something in the case of the woman with the issue of blood who was healed through the healing anointing. It wasn't the healing anointing alone that healed her. Something else was working with the anointing to bring about the healing. What was that something else? It was *faith*.

Jesus said to the woman, "Thy faith hath made thee whole." Some might say, "I thought it was the power which flowed out of Him that made her whole."

Well, really, it was a combination of the two. Both of them—faith and power—are important in their place. Someone who is anointed might minister the power of God, and the anointing may flow through him or her just as electricity flows through a conduit. Yet, although electricity is present all the time, unless someone turns a switch on, there's not going to be any *manifestation* of it.

In the same way, you have to turn the switch of faith on to receive a manifestation of the healing power of God!

Many people have thought that if the power of God was present, it would just manifest itself, regardless of whether or not anyone believed *in* it or believed *for* it. Then if there was no manifestation, they've thought, *Well, the power is not here*. They'd start singing, "Oh, Lord, send the power just now."

Because they couldn't see the anointing or feel it in manifestation, they thought it wasn't there. But the power of God is always present everywhere. God didn't leave most of His power over in one state and then leave only a little bit of it wherever you are! No, wherever God is, *all* of His ability, *all* of His power, *all* of His capabilities are present.

Mixing Faith With the Power

So you can see that it's not a matter of the power getting the job done by itself. No, a person must appropriate or activate the power for himself for it to work for him. Certainly, it's true that it's "*. . . Not by might, nor by power, but by my spirit, saith the Lord . . .*" (Zech. 4:6), but we still have to cooperate with God's Spirit by believing in Him if we want to get the blessing. We've got to learn to mix faith with the power.

Now I tell this story sometimes, and it will further illustrate what I am talking about. In one church I pastored years ago, there was a woman, Sister _____, who had rheumatoid arthritis and was in a wheelchair. Her body had become as stiff as a board. You could take her out of the wheelchair, but you had to hold her and stand her up. She still looked like she was sitting down because her body was frozen in that stationary position.

We had a little prayer group that met every Wednesday afternoon at the church and prayed, and while we were praying one day, I said to the group, "Let's go down to Sister _____'s house and pray for her."

Everyone agreed, so I walked down to Sister _____'s house with my wife and the seven other ladies in the group. We knocked on the door, and Sister _____ invited us in. We talked a little bit, and I said, "Let's pray." I told the ladies to keep their eyes open because I expected Sister _____ to be healed, and I wanted everyone to see it.

Now, as I said earlier, a person can be specially anointed to minister healing—he or she can pray and seek God and minister with that anointing. But, then, you could also, as we sometimes say, "pray the power down." And that's what we did at Sister _____'s house—we prayed until the anointing came into manifestation. Then I pointed to her and said, "Now, my sister, arise and walk in the Name of Jesus!"

The power of God came, and all those ladies, including my wife, are witnesses that Sister _____ rose up out of the chair until she was hovering about two feet above it! And then that same Holy Ghost power brought her forward and she was just suspended in the air.

The Spirit *Upon*

Now if one is anointed with the Spirit, the anointing would flow *through* him, as we saw in Mark chapter 5. The anointing flowed through Jesus to the woman with the issue of blood. But in Sister _____'s case, this anointing came down, as it were, as a result of our *praying*. It came *upon* us.

Sister _____ looked around and saw that she was up above that wheelchair, and she began to whine and cry. She reached back and got hold of the arms of the chair and pulled it up under her. Then she fell back down in it.

Speaking by the Spirit of God, I said, "Sister, you don't have an ounce of faith, do you?" (Of course, I knew she had faith because she was a Spirit-filled Christian. What I was really saying was, "You don't have an ounce of faith when it comes to being healed of rheumatoid arthritis.")

She answered, "No, Brother Hagin, I'll go to my grave from this chair." And, I'm sad to say that she did.

But the power of God was there! It was that power which lifted her up. Now if she had responded to that—if she would have believed it and accepted it—it would have healed her. That's the reason Jesus said in Mark chapter 5, "Daughter, *thy faith* hath made you whole."

The power was there at Sister _____'s house. It didn't come out of me. The anointing was in the room. We were all anointed with the Spirit as we "prayed it down," so to speak.

Prayer Avails Much

The easiest explanation for "praying the power down" comes by reading James 5:16. But let's start with verses 14 and 15.

JAMES 5:14-16
14 Is any sick among you? let him call for the elders of the church; and let them pray over him, anointing him with oil in the name of the Lord:
15 And the prayer of faith shall save the sick, and the Lord shall raise him up; and if he have committed sins, they shall be forgiven him.

16 Confess your faults one to another, and pray one for another, that ye may be healed. The effectual fervent prayer of a righteous man [does a little good. No!] **AVAILETH MUCH.**

The *King James Version* says, "availeth much," but *how* much? I like *The Amplified Bible*, because it tells us how much. It says, ". . . The earnest (heartfelt, continued) prayer of a righteous man makes tremendous power available [dynamic in its working]."

Now notice that the prayer of a righteous man makes *tremendous power* available. This tremendous power is in the spirit realm all the time, isn't it? But the prayer of the righteous makes it *available*. Or, let's say it another way. The prayer of the righteous brings it into *manifestation*.

James says to pray one for another! That means it was scriptural for us to go down and pray for Sister _____. *Pray one for another.* Why? That you may be healed. Then it must be the will of God to heal, or He wouldn't tell us to pray for it.

The effectual fervent prayer of a righteous man availeth much. It makes tremendous power available, dynamic in its action. I like that. Well, you see, we did just what the Scripture said. We went down to Sister _____'s house, and we all prayed. And the power of God came into manifestation.

What was that power that lifted Sister _____ up out of the chair? What was that power that pulled her away from it so that she was sitting in front of it, suspended in the air? It was dynamic Holy Ghost power!

Healing Power Is Always Present

Now, you see, that power is always present. *Power* is always present everywhere, because *God* is always present everywhere.

But just because the power is present doesn't mean it's in manifestation. However, we know from reading James that the effectual fervent prayer of a righteous man makes tremendous power available! Well, we made it available in Sister _____'s case, but that was as far as we could go. We made it available, but she didn't take hold of it.

I couldn't take hold of it for her—I would have if I could have. Jesus *Himself*, couldn't have taken hold of it for her—He would have if He could have. That's the reason He said to the woman with the issue of blood, "Daughter, *thy* faith hath made thee whole."

Even though the power is in manifestation, faith has to be exercised. For it's by faith that we receive any and everything that comes from God.

God moved in a spectacular supernatural way on Sister _____'s behalf. Why wasn't she healed then? What did Jesus say to the woman with the issue of blood? "Daughter, *thy* faith. . . ." Whose faith? *Jesus'* faith? *Peter's* faith? The *apostles'* faith? No! "*THY* faith." It was the *woman's* faith that gave action to God's power!

Remember, God's power is present everywhere! But the fervent effectual prayer of a righteous man makes that tremendous power *available*! That's what we in Pentecostal circles called "praying the power down." But another way to say it is "praying the power into manifestation."

Well, thank God for the Word. And thank God for every avenue of healing: for simple faith in the Word of God; for the laying on of hands by believers and by those specially anointed to minister to the sick; and for supernatural manifestations of the healing power of God. We know that each of these methods of healing is scriptural and that they all work mightily on our behalf—*when we mix faith with the power!*

Questions for Study

1. Name the three ways you can receive healing mentioned in this chapter.

    _____

    _____

2. What are the two ingredients required for each of these methods to work?

    _____

    _____

3. In the spiritual realm, what can you call the thing that turns on the heavenly power?

    _____

    _____

4. Why should we endeavor to preach and teach every side of divine healing?

    _____

    _____

5. It wasn't the healing anointing alone that healed the woman with the issue of blood. What was it that healed her?

    _____

    _____

6. What do you have to do to receive a manifestation of the healing power of God?

    _____

    _____

7. Where does the easiest explanation for "praying the power down" come from?

    _____

    _____

8. Complete this sentence: Even though the power is in _____, faith has to be _____.

9. By what do we receive anything and everything that comes from God?

    _____

    _____

10. When will the three methods of healing mentioned in this chapter work mightily on our behalf?

    _____

    _____

Chapter 17

Faith and Power—Two Ingredients for Receiving Healing—Part 2

In the previous chapter, we began to look at two vital ingredients for receiving healing: *faith* and *power*. I mentioned that there are a number of methods for receiving healing recorded in the Word of God, such as: simple faith; the laying on of hands by believers and by those specially anointed to minister to the sick; and supernatural manifestations of the healing power of God. But I also noted that all of them require *your faith* and *the power of God*.

Remember concerning the power, Acts 10:38 indicates that the terms "the anointing," "the Holy Ghost," and "power" are virtually synonymous. This means that we are able to use them interchangeably when discussing the subject of the healing anointing and the power of God.

Remember that a good analogy for understanding the anointing or the power of God was made by Rev. John G. Lake when he said, *"Electricity is God's power in the natural realm; Holy Ghost power is God's power in the spirit realm."* As I stated previously, just as electricity is in existence in the natural world, the power of God is in existence in the spirit world.

And just as man had to learn how to "plug in" to electricity and make it work for him, we must learn how to "plug in" to the heavenly electricity—the healing power of God—for it to be manifested in our life.

In the natural, when you turn a light switch on, electricity flows right into the lighting fixtures and lights up the room. When you turn the switch off, the lights go out. So in the spiritual realm, the thing that turns on the heavenly power could be called *the switch of faith*!

We've got to learn how to mix *faith* with the *power*!

Let's look at Acts chapter 6, and you'll see that what I'm saying is proven by God's Word.

ACTS 6:3-6

3 Wherefore, brethren, look ye out among you seven men of honest report, full of the Holy Ghost and wisdom, whom we may appoint over this business.

4 But we will give ourselves continually to prayer, and to the ministry of the word.

5 And the saying pleased the whole multitude: and they chose Stephen, a man full of FAITH and of THE HOLY GHOST, and Philip, and Prochorus, and Nicanor, and Timon, and Parmenas, and Nicolas a proselyte of Antioch:

6 Whom they set before the apostles: and when they had prayed, they laid their hands on them.

Just to give you some background and history, here in Acts chapter 6 during the early days of the Church, the believers had "all things in common" (Acts 2:44). The disciples, the twelve apostles, were the only ministers the believers had at the beginning of the Early Church. It was a baby Church, just starting, and the Church didn't exist anywhere except in Jerusalem at that time.

You see, Jesus had said to go into all the world and preach the Gospel to every creature (Mark 16:15). He also said in Acts 1:8 that *". . . after that the Holy Ghost is come upon you . . . ye shall be witnesses unto me both in Jerusalem, and in all Judaea, and in Samaria, and unto the uttermost part of the earth."* Yet the believers hadn't witnessed to anyone anywhere except in Jerusalem.

So there in Jerusalem, the believers had all things in common, but some of them felt as though they were being neglected in the daily ministrations. So the Twelve said, *"Wherefore, brethren, look ye out among you seven men of HONEST REPORT, FULL OF THE HOLY GHOST and WISDOM, whom we may appoint over this business"* (Acts 6:3).

The men they were looking for had to meet three requirements. They had to: 1) have an honest report; 2) be full of the Holy Ghost; and 3) be full of wisdom.

Full of Faith and Power

Verse 5 goes on to list the seven men who were chosen to oversee the daily ministrations. Now all seven of these men were full of the Holy Ghost.

That was one of the qualifications—that they be full of the Holy Ghost. But it says about Stephen that he was full of faith *and* the Holy Ghost or power. And there were certain miracles and signs that followed Stephen's mix of faith and power.

ACTS 6:8
8   And Stephen, FULL OF FAITH AND POWER, did great wonders and miracles among the people.

You see, if you are full of the Holy Ghost, you're full of power. I mean, you've got the Powerhouse in you! Well, every one of those seven men were full of power. But that doesn't mean that every one of them was full of faith.

Did you ever stop to think about the fact that every Spirit-filled believer—every believer who maintains the Spirit-filled experience—is full of power. He doesn't have to *get* full; he *is* full.

Now to be filled with the Spirit is to be filled with power. Jesus said in Acts 1:8, *"But ye shall receive POWER, after that the HOLY GHOST is come upon you. . . ."*

So we read in Acts 6:3 that the apostles said, *". . . look ye out among you seven men of honest report, FULL OF THE HOLY GHOST* [power] *and wisdom, whom we may appoint over this business."*

All seven men listed in Acts 6:5 were full of the Holy Ghost. That means that all seven of these men were full of *power*. But apparently, there was only one of them who did any miracles and signs among the people, and that was Stephen.

Every one of them had the power to do the miracles and signs. Why didn't they do them then? *Because it takes faith to give action to the power!*

Faith Activates the Power

You can see where we as Spirit-filled believers and Pentecostal people, particularly in days gone by, have missed it. We've thought that if we had the power, the miracles and the wonders would just automatically follow.

But they won't. We saw that in Acts chapter 6. All seven of those men were full of power, but only one of them did any miracles or wonders, and that was Stephen. And Stephen wasn't even one of the Twelve. He wasn't a preacher or an apostle or an evangelist. In fact, according to the Scripture, he never did become an evangelist or an apostle or pastor; he lived and died a deacon.

ACTS 6:8
8   And Stephen, full of faith and power, did great wonders and miracles among the people.

Stephen didn't do great wonders and miracles just by being full of power. No, he was full of faith *and* power. And so we know that power by itself won't get the job done. You have to mix faith *with* the power to get the power to work.

Did you notice that the same thing is true in the case of an individual's healing? For example, in the case of the woman with the issue of blood, Jesus knew immediately that power had gone out of Him. But He didn't say, "Daughter, My *power* hath made thee whole." No, He said, "Daughter, thy *faith* hath made thee whole" (Mark 5:34). It was her faith mixed with the power that healed her.

Faith Comes by Hearing

Also, notice that when Jesus and His disciples crossed over the Sea of Galilee to the land of Gennesaret in Matthew chapter 14, the people of that place "had knowledge of Jesus" and brought the sick and diseased to Him. As the sick and the diseased touched the hem of Jesus' garment, they were made whole (vv. 35,36).

But notice the men of Gennesaret did that *when* they "had knowledge of Him." They had to have heard about Jesus to have knowledge of Him. Well, we know that "faith comes by hearing, and hearing by the Word of God" (Rom. 10:17). So again, faith was involved.

Then in Luke chapter 6, it says the multitude came to hear Jesus and to be healed of their diseases. It said they sought to touch Jesus, for there went virtue or power out of Him and healed them all. But notice they came to *hear* and to be healed. They heard *first*, then faith came, and then they sought to touch Him.

People need to understand the healing anointing. They need to know that it exists, but just as importantly, they need to know how to get that anointing to work and produce results in their lives. They need to believe or have faith in the healing power of God.

Sometimes, the healing power of God is ministered to a sick person so that the person is manifestly supercharged with heavenly electricity. *Yet no real or final healing takes place until something occurs that releases the faith of the individual.*

After I started preaching, I would teach people faith. Once in a while, we'd have manifestations of the Spirit or the anointing, and folks would receive healing as a result of their faith mixed with the power of God. But I'd see a lot of people healed when we didn't feel anything. We just believed, and it happened!

Yet, right on the other hand, even back then, people I'd pray for would say sometimes, "Something's all over me!" Well, I knew they were talking about the same thing that happened to me when I was healed. And those people were healed, because the Spirit was present! And they mixed faith with the power and were healed!

Manifested Power

Now I want to show you something about mixing faith with the power to receive healing. When I was young and the new pastor of a Full Gospel church in northcentral Texas, we had just moved into the parsonage and were unloading boxes and straightening things up.

There was a knock on the parsonage door. I went to the door and there stood a little cotton-headed boy. Now someone asked me, "What do you mean, 'cotton-headed'?" Well, I just mean his hair was white like cotton. He was about nine years old. He said, "Momma wants you to come and pray for her."

I said, "Who's momma?" because I didn't know him—I had only been the pastor for two Sundays. I hadn't gotten acquainted with everyone yet.

The little boy told me his momma's name, and I recognized her as being one of the Sunday school teachers. So I said, "Son, stand right there. I'll put on my tie and coat, and you can show me the way to go because I don't know where you live."

I took the little bottle of anointing oil that I had, and we went to the little boy's house. I anointed this boy's momma with oil, laid hands on her, prayed, and got up to leave.

She said, "Brother B_____ [and she gave the name of the former pastor] always prayed till the power fell."

I knew that the power of God does "fall" because the Bible said that while Peter yet spake unto them, the Holy Ghost fell on them (Acts 10:44). And Acts 8 also refers to the Holy Ghost this way.

ACTS 8:14-16
14 Now when the apostles which were at Jerusalem heard that Samaria had received the word of God, they sent unto them Peter and John:
15 Who, when they were come down, prayed for them, that they might receive the Holy Ghost:
16 (For as yet he was FALLEN UPON none of them. . . .)

That's the part I want you to get. The Holy Ghost *does* fall on people—like rain. In fact, the latter rain is a type of the Holy Ghost.

'Praying the Power Down'

Back in 1939, I didn't know exactly what to do when she said "pray the power down" because I was new in Pentecostal circles. I didn't know how they did things. But I figured if that was the way the former pastor did it, then that was the way to do it. So I got back down on my knees and prayed till the power fell. It took me an hour and a half, but I prayed the power down! The house shook, the bed shook, and the woman shook.

It was summertime—the sky was blue with just a few white clouds. There wasn't a leaf stirring on any tree. And yet the windows rattled!

Well, I got up off my knees and went home to the parsonage.

That afternoon there was a knock on the parsonage door. I went to the door and there stood that little cotton-headed boy. He said, "Momma wants you to come and pray for her."

I said, "I thought she got healed this morning."

He said, "She did, but she's worse now."

So I went down there and prayed the power down again—the power fell, she shook, the bed shook, the house shook, and the windows shook. So I went back to the parsonage.

The next day there was another knock on the door. I went to the door, and there stood that little cotton-headed boy. He said, "Momma wants you to come and pray for her."

I said, "I thought she got healed twice yesterday."

"Well, she did, but she's hurting worse today."

So I went down there again and prayed the power down. By that time, I was becoming an expert at praying the power down, so it didn't take an hour and a half to pray it down. I did it in an hour, and then I went home.

The next day there was a knock on the door, so I went to the door, and there stood that cotton-headed boy! The same scenario happened again and again until I finally got to where I could pray the power down in thirty minutes. She shook, the bed shook, the windows rattled, and the house shook. And that went on, and on, and on.

If you think I'm exaggerating, we'll skip ahead to three years later. This went on for three years! We had been building onto the parsonage, and there was a little work left to finish. I worked a little late on it one night because I didn't want to have to work the next day. After I finished, I was getting ready for church because we were having revival that night. As I was quickly getting ready, I heard my wife let someone in the house. I looked up, and there was that cotton-headed boy.

Now he and I had been working together so long that we knew what the other was thinking.

So I said, before he could say it, "Yeah, I know, momma wants me to come and pray for her."

When the cotton-headed boy arrived, it was only about ten minutes until the church service was supposed to start. (The parsonage was right next door, so I still had plenty of time to get to the church.)

I was about to say, "Will it be all right to come after church?" I had just started to speak when he said, "No, she said to come before church. She's hurting awfully bad!"

I wondered how in the world I was going to get down there, pray the power down, get back, and start church in ten minutes. I quickly put my tie and coat on.

I had a car, but I knew I could get there faster by going down the back alley. So I ran out of the parsonage, ran behind the church, down one alley, back up another alley, across the street, down another alley, and knocked on the door.

She told me to come in. I had my bottle of oil out before I even got in the door. I went in and anointed her with oil. I said, "Oh, God, heal this woman in the Name of Jesus. You said if we'd ask in Your Name, You'd do it, so You've done it. Amen." That's exactly what I said, and I said it double time!

I put the top on my bottle of oil and headed for the door—I had to go back and start church! She started to say something, but I said, "I know, Sister, you're hurting worse now than you did when I came in here a few seconds ago. But you're healed, and the next time I see you, you'll tell me it's so." And I ran out and slammed the door.

I ran up one alley, across the street, up another alley, behind the church, and went in through a side door. I looked at my watch—it was exactly time to start. We started church, sang, took up an offering for the evangelist, and made the announcements.

Just before the evangelist was going to speak, I said, "Let's have about three testimonies, one from each section. Someone who has been saved, healed, or baptized with the Holy Ghost during this revival, stand up and give your testimony."

So one person stood and testified. Then another one from a different section stood and testified. About that time, the double doors in the back of the church opened. And this lady, Sister S_____, who'd been having me pray the power down for *three years*, came in. I guess she thought we were having a testimony meeting, because she came down the aisle waving her arms and said, "It's just like you said, Brother Hagin. You hadn't been gone ten minutes when every pain and every symptom left me."

Hallelujah! I pastored that woman nearly eighteen more months and never did have to go pray for her again!

Keeping Your Healing

Thank God for the power. But remember this, if you don't believe God—the power can shake the house and everything else, and *still* nothing will happen to *you*. This lady received her healing and finally *kept* it because she believed God herself.

The reason I tell this story is to show that although the healing power may be ministered to a person, and though that person may manifestly be supercharged with the power of God, no real and final healing will take place until something occurs that releases the faith of the individual.

The Bible says in Hebrews 4:2, *"For unto us was the gospel preached, as well as unto them* [talking about Israel]*: but the word preached did not profit them, NOT BEING MIXED WITH FAITH in them that heard it."*

One way to receive the healing power, of course, is through the laying on of hands (Mark 16:18).

Or you could receive it from a cloth or a handkerchief that has absorbed the anointing (Acts 19:11-12). On the other hand, receiving healing that way is only *one* way to receive. Remember I said you could receive healing by acting in simple faith on the Word of God, as I did to receive my healing (Mark 11:22-24).

The Holy Ghost is ever-present with all the power He has! You can mix your faith with the power that is present, whether the power is in manifestation or not, and receive your healing by faith.

In conclusion, let's sum up a few things about the healing power of God. When we understand some things about the anointing, we can appropriate it for ourselves and reap the benefit of this power in our own lives.

The healing anointing is a tangible substance. And the Word of God reveals to us the rules and laws that govern its operation.

The Lord Jesus Christ revealed and applied the laws of the Spirit, which demonstrated the fact that the healing power of God is a tangible substance, a heavenly materiality.

Now you'll not receive any of this power from Heaven if you don't believe there's any there. If you don't believe it exists, you'll never get it applied to your circumstances so that it will do you any good. The healing power of God will not benefit you until you believe in it, lay hold of it intelligently by faith, and simply receive it.

But, thank God, through your faith in the holy written Word and in the mighty power of God, you *can* receive divine healing! By believing what God's Word says about the healing anointing, you can enjoy all the blessings and benefits of this power from Heaven that is available to us today.

Questions for Study

1. We've got to learn how to mix _____ with the power.

2. If you are filled with the Holy Ghost, what are you full of?

   _____

   _____

3. According to Romans 10:17, how does faith come?

   _____

   _____

4. In Luke chapter 6, what two things did the multitude come to do?

   _____

   _____

5. What two things do people need to know concerning the healing anointing?

   _____

   _____

6. No real or final healing takes place until what happens?

   _____

   _____

7. What are two ways the healing power can be received or transferred?

   _____

   _____

8. How must faith be released?

   _____

   _____

9. What reveals to us the rules and laws that govern the operation of the healing power of God?

   _____

   _____

10. The healing power of God will not benefit you until you do what three things?

   _____

   _____

Chapter 18

The Gifts of the Spirit

We are discussing biblical ways to receive healing. There are many different methods listed in the Bible whereby you can receive healing. One way to receive healing is through the manifestation of one of the gifts of the Spirit.

The nine gifts of the Spirit listed in First Corinthians 12:8-10 are often divided into three separate categories, because they naturally seem to fit there. Any one of the nine gifts may be used, as the Spirit wills, to aid in the area of healing. The most common spiritual gifts used concerning healing are the power gifts: the working of miracles, the gift of faith, and the gifts of healing. And these "power" gifts will very often work together.

Working of miracles is defined as a divine intervention in the ordinary course of nature that can't be explained in the natural. For example, the dividing of a stream by the sweep of a mantle is an example of the working of miracles in operation (2 Kings 2:14). After Elijah ascended into Heaven in a chariot in the whirlwind, Elisha received his mantle and smote the Jordan River. Dividing the waters by a sweep of his mantle was the working of miracles because that was a supernatural intervention in the ordinary course of nature.

In the area of healing, many times miracles are received. However this is not necessarily the working of miracles but is simply called healing miracles. Everything that God does is miraculous, in a sense, but receiving healing by supernatural means is not a miracle in the same sense that turning common dust into insects just by a gesture is a miracle (Exod. 8:16), or turning common water into wine just by speaking a word is a miracle (John 2:7-11). Those two occurrences are examples of the working of miracles.

Although in the Old Testament people were healed and the gifts of healings were in operation, gifts of healings were more commonly in operation in the New Testament than they were in the Old Testament.

On the other hand, the working of miracles was more prominent or more commonly manifested in the Old Testament than in the New Testament, with the exception of the gift of working of miracles in Jesus' ministry.

The Gift of Faith

Now I want to focus on the gift of faith. I like the *Weymouth* translation of First Corinthians 12:9, because it calls this spiritual gift "special faith." You see, this faith is *special* faith because every believer already has faith (Rom. 12:3).

For example, there is *saving* faith, or faith to receive salvation, which is also a gift of God.

EPHESIANS 2:8
8   For by grace are ye SAVED THROUGH FAITH; and that not of yourselves: it is the gift of God.

The faith by which you are saved is a gift of God, but it is given to you through hearing the Word. The Bible says, *"So then faith* [saving faith] *cometh by hearing, and hearing by the WORD OF GOD"* (Rom. 10:17). But the gift of faith is distinct from saving faith. It is a supernatural manifestation of one of the nine gifts of the Spirit.

The gift of faith is a gift of the Spirit to the believer that he might *receive* a miracle, whereas the working of miracles is a gift of the Spirit to the believer that he might *work* a miracle. (One gift *receives* something, and the other *does* something.) But these gifts are very closely related. We're just differentiating between them for the purpose of defining them.

So then, we said that the *gift of faith* is separate and distinct from *saving faith*. It is also distinct from the *fruit* of faith that we're taught about in the New Testament.

GALATIANS 5:22
22 . . . the fruit of the Spirit is love, joy, peace, long-suffering, gentleness, goodness, FAITH.

Galatians 5:22 says that faith is a fruit of the spirit. However, if you look up this word in the original Greek translation, you will find that it refers to *faithfulness*.

The fruit of the spirit are for *character*, but the gifts of the Spirit are for *power*. A fruit is something that grows. So faith, or faithfulness, is a spiritual fruit that grows in the life of the Christian to establish him in spiritual character. The *gift of faith*, however, is given supernaturally by the Spirit of God, as He wills (1 Cor. 12:11).

So you can see that there are different kinds of faith. Saving faith comes before salvation, and the fruit of faith comes or develops after salvation. But the manifestation of the gift of faith comes after the baptism in the Holy Spirit, as the Spirit wills.

Many times people—even Christians—who haven't studied the Bible say, "Well, if God gives me faith, I'll have it. And if He doesn't, I won't." They read in First Corinthians 12:9, "to another is given faith," and they may think that's how all faith works. But that verse is talking about the gift of faith, which is separate from all other kinds of faith. The gift of faith is a gift of the Spirit to the believer that he might receive a miracle!

Remember, the working of miracles employs faith that actively *works* a miracle. But the gift of faith employs faith that passively *expects* a miracle as a sustained or continuous action. There may not be anything that the person sees at the moment to confirm that he has his answer. But special faith will carry over a long period of time. In other words, its manifestation can be sustained or continued for the purpose of receiving a miracle.

A Supernatural Endowment

The gift of faith is also a supernatural endowment by the Holy Spirit whereby that which is uttered or desired by man, or spoken by God, eventually comes to pass. In other words, when this power gift is in operation, you believe God in such a way that God honors your word as His own and miraculously brings to pass whatever you believe or say. So the miracle, utterance, assurance, curse or blessing, creation or destruction, or removal or alteration has to manifest when it has been spoken under the inspiration of this gift.

In my own life, I've always been one to believe God's Word and act upon it. But I'm conscious of times when special faith is operating in my life. And it doesn't bother me a bit in the world whether or not I see anything. I'll just laugh right in the face of the circumstances, because I know that the Word has been spoken, and it shall to come to pass!

Faith To Raise the Dead

Smith Wigglesworth said that if you will take a step of faith—use the measure of faith you have as a Christian—when you come to the end of that faith, very often this supernatural gift of special faith will take over.

Under Wigglesworth's ministry, at least three different people were raised from the dead. In his book *Ever Increasing Faith*, Wigglesworth related one instance of his neighbor being raised from the dead.[1]

One day Wigglesworth visited a sick neighbor who had been close to death. After coming home from an open-air meeting the following day, Wigglesworth learned that his wife Polly was at this neighbor's house. As Wigglesworth approached the house, he heard screaming. He went inside and found the sick man's wife, crying, "He's gone! He's gone!"

Wigglesworth said, "I just passed by the man's wife and went into the room. Immediately, I saw that he was gone. I could not understand it, but I began to pray. My wife was always afraid that I would go too far, and she laid hold of me and said, 'Don't, Dad! Don't you see that he is dead?' But I continued praying.

"I got as far as I could with my own faith, and then God laid hold of me. It was such a laying hold that I could believe for anything. The faith of the Lord Jesus laid hold of me, and a solid peace came into my heart. I shouted, 'He lives! He lives! He lives!' And my neighbor is still living today."

Well, you know as well as I do, that receiving the dead back to life is beyond anyone's ordinary faith. In our ordinary faith, we could pull a dead person off his deathbed, stand him up, and tell him to walk. But that doesn't mean he would begin to walk. Why not? Because it would take a miracle—and it takes a supernatural manifestation of God's power to receive a miracle from God!

As I said before, the working of miracles *performs* a miracle, but the gift of faith *receives* a miracle. So the working of miracles is more of an *act*, whereas the gift of faith is more of a *process*.

We can see that by the gift of faith, the miraculous was manifested in the Scriptures. People were supernaturally fed and sustained. Angels stood guard over and protected the servants of God. Men were delivered from the ferocity of beasts. And the dead were raised to life. But the *present-day* use of this power gift is still the same.

In the same way that the gift of faith was manifested in Bible days, it can be manifested to receive supernatural blessings, protection, or sustenance today. By this power gift, evil spirits can be cast out and the dead can be raised. But it takes supernatural faith—special faith—for those things to happen!

The Gifts Work Together

As I have mentioned, the three power gifts—the working of miracles, the gift of faith, and the gifts of healings—will very often work together. In the case of raising the dead, all three of these power gifts operate together.

First of all, in raising the dead, it takes supernatural faith—the gift of special faith—to call a person's spirit back after it has left the body. Then it takes the working of miracles because the body would have started to deteriorate, as in the case of Lazarus (John 11:39).

And then raising the dead also takes the gifts of healings because if the person who was raised from the dead wasn't healed, whatever he died from would still affect his body and he would die again. So the person would have

to be healed too. Therefore, all three of the power gifts are in manifestation when someone is raised from the dead.

Gifts of Healings

We have looked at the "power" gifts of the Spirit—the gifts that *do* something—mentioned in First Corinthians 12:9 and 10. We have discussed the *working of miracles* and the *gift of faith*. Now I want to focus on the *gifts of healings*.

In the original Greek translation of First Corinthians 12:9 and 30, this gift is listed as "gifts of healings"—both *gifts* and *healings* are plural. Therefore, we will refer to this spiritual gift as the *gifts of healings*.

As we study the gifts of healings in Scripture, we see that they are manifested for the supernatural healing of diseases and infirmities without natural means of any sort.

For example, Luke, the writer of the Acts of the Apostles and the Gospel that bears his name, was a medical doctor by profession. He accompanied Paul on many missionary journeys and was traveling with him when they were shipwrecked on the island of Melita. When we read the account in Acts 28, nothing is ever said about Luke ministering to anyone while they were there. But the Bible says that Paul ministered to several on the island who were sick or had diseases, and they were healed. How? By the supernatural power of God!

ACTS 28:8,9
8   And it came to pass, that the father of Publius lay sick of a fever and of a bloody flux: to whom PAUL ENTERED IN, AND PRAYED, AND LAID HIS HANDS ON HIM, AND HEALED HIM.
9   So when this was done, OTHERS ALSO, WHICH HAD DISEASES IN THE ISLAND, CAME, AND WERE HEALED.

Now some have mistakenly thought that the gifts of healings refer to the fact that God has given us doctors and medical science. Of course, we believe in medical science and doctors, and thank God for what they can do—we are certainly not opposed to them. But the gifts of the

Spirit are *supernatural*. They have nothing to do with medical science.

Healing that is supernatural doesn't come by a diagnosis and the prescribing of treatment. It comes by the laying on of hands, anointing with oil, or sometimes just speaking God's Word in faith! So we not only believe in *natural* healing, but we also believe in *supernatural* healing!

How Jesus Ministered

The Bible is full of examples of the gifts of healings in operation—delivering the sick and destroying the works of the devil in a person's human body—especially through Jesus' ministry. However, I often point out the fact that Jesus ministered as a prophet anointed by the Holy Ghost.

Notice, for instance, what Jesus said of Himself in the synagogue, reading from the Prophet Isaiah: *"The Spirit of the Lord is upon me, because HE HATH ANOINTED ME . . ."* (Luke 4:18). Then in Acts 10:38, Peter said, *". . . GOD ANOINTED JESUS of Nazareth with the Holy Ghost and with power: who went about doing good, and healing all. . . ."*

Jesus never healed anyone until *after* He was anointed with the Holy Ghost and power. And yet He was just as much the Son of God when He was twenty-five years old as He was at age thirty. So Jesus didn't heal the sick by some power that was inherent in Him as the Second Person of the Trinity. He healed them the same way anyone else would minister to the sick today—by the anointing of the Spirit or the manifestation of the gifts of healings!

Now the main thing we need to understand is that there is a difference between the manifestation of the gifts of healings and receiving healing by one's own faith in God's Word.

When I teach, I emphasize that people can receive healing simply by exercising faith in the Word of God—because it always works. Many of you know my testimony of how I received healing as a young Baptist boy reading Grandma's Methodist Bible. I wasn't healed because I believed in

divine healing, necessarily. I was healed by *acting* and *standing* on Mark 11:24!

I read in Mark 11:24 that Jesus said, *". . .What things soever ye DESIRE, when ye pray, believe that ye receive them, and ye shall have them."* Well, I desired healing. So I prayed and began to say: "I believe I receive healing for my deformed heart, I believe I receive healing for my paralyzed body, I believe I receive healing for my incurable blood condition," and so forth.

To make a long story short, God's healing power was manifested in my body. No one laid hands on me. That power came unto me directly from God. But when the *gifts of healings* are in operation, they're manifested *through another person* unto you, as the Spirit wills. That's the difference. The healing always comes from God, however.

Healing as a Gift vs. Gifts of Healings

Now some have said, "Any time you receive healing, it's a manifestation of the gifts of healings." But I disagree with that statement. Healing is a gift, all right, in the general sense that anything you receive from God would be a gift. But that doesn't necessarily mean that these spiritual gifts are in operation. For example, that wasn't the case when I received healing as a young boy on the bed of sickness.

Others have taken this reasoning one step further, saying, "Healing is a gift. So anytime you get healed, *you* have received a gift of healing." But I can't accept that explanation either, because it doesn't line up with Scripture. Take a look at First Corinthians 12:28-30.

1 CORINTHIANS 12:28-30
28 And GOD HATH SET SOME IN THE CHURCH, first apostles, secondarily prophets, thirdly teachers, after that miracles, THEN GIFTS OF HEALINGS, helps, governments, diversities of tongues.
29 Are all apostles? are all prophets? are all teachers? are all workers of miracles?
30 HAVE ALL THE GIFTS OF HEALING [healings] **. . .?**

Notice in verse 28 that God set "some" in the Church. Paul isn't talking about spiritual gifts, because he said in verse 27, *"Now ye are the body of Christ, and MEMBERS in particular."*

No, Paul is referring to men equipped with spiritual gifts. God set *members equipped with spiritual gifts* in the Church—first, apostles; secondarily, prophets; thirdly, teachers; and so forth.

You see, the "gift" of the apostle, prophet, or teacher is a ministry gift given to the Church, not an individual gift that someone might receive (Eph. 4:8,11). In other words, it's not given to bless *you*! It's given in order to bless *others*. It's a ministry!

First Corinthians 12:28 goes on to say, "*after that* miracles," meaning: "*After those who are equipped with the ministry gifts which Paul just mentioned*, there are some in the ministry who are equipped with the gift of the working of miracles." (A better way to say it would be that the gift of the working of miracles operates by the Spirit more consistently in some people's ministries.)

Next Paul mentions the gifts of healings, and he asks a few rhetorical questions: "Does everyone have the ministry of an apostle?" Certainly not. "Does everyone have the ministry of a prophet?" No. "Does everyone have the ministry of the teacher?" No. We could all teach to some extent, of course. But there are those whom God has put in the Church who are specifically equipped or anointed by the Holy Spirit with a teaching gift.

So, you see, the gifts of healings are not referring to gifts given to individuals to bless them personally. They are *ministries* of healing that are given to some in order to bless others. I like to say it this way: The gifts of healings are supernatural manifestations of the Spirit that are manifested *through someone* to *someone else*!

Laying On of Hands

When I started out in the healing ministry as a Baptist boy preacher, I wasn't conscious of any kind of anointing or special manifestation of the Spirit. I just prayed for people in faith through the laying on of hands and anointing with oil. I received the baptism in the Holy Ghost later, but I continued to pray for the sick the same way.

Then in 1938, I accepted the pastorate of a little Full Gospel church in the blacklands of northcentral Texas, where I met my wife Oretha. After we were married, Oretha and I lived with her folks, who owned a large farmhouse. Neither she nor her parents had received the baptism in the Holy Ghost yet, so when we all gathered to pray, I did my best to behave myself.

But one night we got to praying and I unconsciously started praying in tongues right out loud. I prayed in tongues approximately 45 minutes, and then the Spirit of God said to me, "Lay your hand on your wife, and I'll fill her with the Holy Ghost." So I reached out my hand and laid it on top of Oretha's head.

Oretha had never sought the Holy Ghost a minute in her life, but the second I laid my hand on her head, she threw up both hands and started talking in tongues instantly. She never stammered or stuttered. She just began speaking fluently in other tongues as the Spirit of the Lord gave her utterance.

Special Anointing

Well, that same night around midnight, the Lord ministered to me by His Spirit concerning the gifts of healings and His sending me out to minister to the sick. Now as I said, I would anoint people with oil and lay hands on them for healing, simply praying with them in faith. In other words, none of the gifts of the Spirit were in operation. God's healing power would manifest itself directly unto *them*.

But on occasion I would be conscious of a manifestation of God's power working through *me*. That didn't always happen (it was as the Spirit willed), but I was aware of it when it did. I really didn't do a whole lot about it, though, except yield to the Spirit of God.

Ten years later I was pastoring a church in east Texas, and I started to become dissatisfied spiritually. Naturally speaking, I had every cause in the world to feel good and rejoice. Folks had been getting saved, filled with the Spirit, and healed in the church. But I was just flat dissatisfied.

So I spent some concentrated time shut up in the church, praying, reading my Bible, and seeking God about ministry. While I was at the altar praying one day, the Lord asked me: "What are you going to do about the healing ministry and what I said to you ten years ago in that little farmhouse in northcentral Texas?"

I said, "To tell You the truth, Lord, I didn't intend to do anything about it."

He said, "You're going to have to—or else."

Well, I had run into some of the Lord's "or else's" through the years, so I said to Him, "Yes, Sir! I believe I will." And I left the last church I pastored in February 1949 to go out into field ministry and endeavor to do what God had called me to do.

Heart Trouble

One night while holding a meeting in a Full Gospel church in Henderson, Texas, I was praying for the sick by the laying on of hands. A woman from the church came up, and the Spirit of God gave me a word of knowledge concerning her: "Thy heart is not right with God."

I knew I should have spoken that word out, but I was reluctant. (That's a terrible thing to have to tell someone.) So I bit my tongue and shut my mouth to keep from saying anything. And, suddenly, the anointing lifted from me like a cloud and floated away.

I had been staying in the parsonage as the pastor's guest, and the minute I lay down to go to sleep that night, it felt as if my heart just stopped. I reached up to feel my chest and couldn't feel any heartbeat, just a faint fluttering or shaking. I rolled out of bed and hit the cold linoleum floor, yelling at the top of my voice: "Lord, I'll obey You next time! I'll do what You want me to do!" I was so loud that I woke the pastor and his wife in their bedroom at the opposite end of the house!

I made my way to the dining room and called out to the pastor to come pray for me. As death fastened its final throes on me, I could feel myself slipping out of my body. I'd had the same experience twice before, so I knew that death had come.

I wanted to leave a word for the pastor to tell my wife and children. But when I opened my mouth to speak, I began to prophesy instead. I had never done much prophesying before, but I started to prophesy out of my spirit—and God began to speak to me through my own words.

You see, I had not fully obeyed Him in some areas concerning the gifts of the Spirit, because I was afraid what people would think. I thought they'd think I was trying to attract attention to myself if I ministered the way He was leading me when His gifts were in manifestation.

But the Spirit of the Lord said to me: "When Peter and John saw the man who was crippled at the gate called Beautiful, Peter stopped and said to him, 'Look on us!' " (Acts 3:4).

ACTS 3:2-6
2 And a certain man lame from his mother's womb was carried, whom they laid daily at the gate of the temple which is called Beautiful . . . ;
3 Who seeing Peter and John about to go into the temple asked an alms.
4 And Peter, fastening his eyes upon him with John, said, LOOK ON US.
5 And he gave heed unto them, EXPECTING TO RECEIVE SOMETHING OF THEM.
6 Then Peter said, Silver and gold have I none; but such as I have give I thee: In the name of Jesus Christ of Nazareth rise up and walk.

Expectancy

As I continued to speak out of my spirit, the Lord explained: "Peter didn't say that to draw attention to John and himself or to brag about something they had. He said it in order to raise the man's expectancy—so that he would expect to receive what Peter and John had from God" (v. 5)!

Then the Spirit of the Lord said to me, "It wouldn't have done any good for Peter to say, 'The gifts of healings are in operation,' because the man wouldn't have known anything about that. The New Testament had not yet been written."

The Spirit of the Lord continued, "You see, people can be healed directly from Me because they believe and exercise faith in the promises of God, just as you did. But many people are not at the place spiritually where they can receive healing on their own. Therefore, I want you to tell them that I have anointed you and sent you to minister to the sick.

"When you do that, you're not attracting attention to yourself, you're arousing the people's expectancy. If you can just arouse their expectancy, they wouldn't need any more faith than just to expect Me to heal them *through* you as My gifts are in manifestation."

I saw the difference then. And that's what I want to get over to you. *You can be healed directly, simply by believing God—and I believe that's the best way to receive healing.* But everyone is not going to receive that way. That's why we need to pray along these lines.

Pray what? That all would have the gifts of healings? No, we already saw in First Corinthians chapter 12 that not everyone will have the gifts of healings operating through them. But thank God, *some will!*

Well, thank God for the privilege to believe and act on God's Word. We should be doing that continually. But we can also pray that the gifts of healings would be supernaturally manifested among us even more, and expect God's power to flow unto others *through* members of His Body, as the Spirit wills!

_____

[1]Smith Wigglesworth, *Ever Increasing Faith*, (Springfield, Missouri: Gospel Publishing House, 1971), pp. 138,139.

Questions for Study

1. Which group of spiritual gifts are most commonly used concerning healing?

   _____

   _____

2. List these three "power" gifts.

   _____

   _____

3. What kind of faith is used to receive salvation?

   _____

   _____

4. What is the gift of faith?

   _____

   _____

5. Complete this sentence: The fruit of the spirit are for _____, but the gifts of the Spirit are for _____.

6. What did Jesus minister as?

   _____

   _____

7. Where does healing always come from?

   _____

   _____

8. What are gifts of healings?

   _____

   _____

9. According to Acts 3:5, when the man gave heed unto Peter and John, what was he expecting?

   _____

   _____

10. We can act and believe on God's Word, and we should be doing that continually. But what else can we be doing?

    _____

    _____

Chapter 19

The Healing Anointing

In previous chapters, we discussed how faith will activate the healing power of God. You can activate the healing power by your own faith in the Word of God, as I did on the eighth day of August, 1934. By faith, I "plugged in" to the healing power of God that was present in my room and was raised up from the bed of sickness.

We have also discussed how you can receive healing by the laying on of hands. We know this method is scriptural because we are told in Mark's Gospel to lay hands on the sick (Mark 16:18). Any believer can lay hands on the sick based on this particular verse of Scripture. But there are also those who are specially anointed to minister healing to the sick.

In this chapter, I want to further discuss the healing anointing, with a focus on the ways the anointing may be transferred by a person specially anointed to minister healing.

As I said in a previous chapter, Acts 10:38 indicates that the terms,"the anointing," "the Holy Ghost," and "power" are virtually synonymous. This means that we are able to use these terms interchangeably when discussing the subject of the healing anointing and the power of God.

Concerning the individual anointing, we know that God anoints individuals to minister. There are different offices in which God calls them to minister—the office of the apostle, prophet, evangelist, pastor, and teacher. Jesus stood in all five of them, so He had the anointing that goes with every office.

Jesus had the anointing *without measure* (John 3:34). Members of the Body of Christ have the anointing *in a measure.*

Of course, Jesus was and is the Son of God. But Jesus was not *ministering* as the Son of God. He was *ministering* as a mere man anointed with the Holy Ghost! If Jesus was ministering on the earth as the Son of God and not as a man, then He wouldn't need to be anointed. But the Bible plainly says Jesus was anointed to minister on the earth (Luke 4:18; Acts 10:38).

Characteristics of the Healing Anointing

I want to look at some characteristics of the anointing, which will help you understand the way it works. First, the anointing is *transmittable.*

MATTHEW 14:35,36
35 And when the men of that place had knowledge of him [Jesus], they sent out into all that country round about, and brought unto him all that were diseased;
36 And besought him that they might only touch the HEM of his garment: and as many as touched were made perfectly whole.

You'll notice that in Matthew chapter 14, those people sought to touch the hem of Jesus' garment. They didn't touch *Him*; they just touched the hem of His *garment*, and they were healed!

Then in Mark's Gospel, we read that the woman with the issue of blood *". . . came in the press behind, and touched his [Jesus'] garment"* (Mark 5:27). Well, evidently, Jesus' garment became charged with that same power or anointing with which He Himself was anointed.

Also, the cloths that Paul laid hands upon became charged with the same anointing that Paul was anointed with, which was the healing and delivering power of God (Acts 19:11,12).

Then it seems that the healing power of God can be absorbed by certain materials, namely cloths. And that healing power or anointing can be transmitted or transferred from the cloths into the bodies of the sick.

The anointing is also measurable. We read in the Old Testament that God commanded the prophet Elijah to anoint Elisha to take his place, and it says Elisha asked for a double portion of Elijah's anointing (2 Kings 2:9).

Then in the Gospels we saw that Jesus was anointed to minister as He walked upon the earth. And John 3:34 says that Jesus had the anointing *without measure*.

The anointing is also *tangible*. The word "tangible" means *perceptible to the touch*. In other words, something that is tangible is capable of being touched.

For example, we know that the anointing that went into the woman with the issue of blood in Mark chapter 5 was tangible because Jesus knew *immediately* when that power went out of Him. Jesus was aware of an *outflow* of that healing power, and the woman was aware of the *reception* of that power. So the power had to have been tangible.

Ways the Anointing Is Transferred

Now that we've looked at the characteristics of the healing anointing, I want to focus on the ways it is transferred. One way is by the laying on of hands.

In His own ministry, Jesus used many methods in ministering to the sick. Sometimes He just said, "Arise and walk," and they arose and walked. But one of the main ways He ministered healing was by the laying on of hands.

For example, in Mark chapter 5, Jesus laid hands on Jairus' daughter, and she was healed. All through the New Testament, there are a number of instances where Jesus laid His hands on the sick and they were healed. The contact of His hands with the sick one permitted the healing anointing, or the power of God in Him, to flow into the sick one.

The healing anointing can also be transferred, as I mentioned earlier, through a cloth, such as a garment or handkerchief.

In Mark chapter 5, the woman with the issue of blood touched Jesus' clothes and found the power of God emanating from His Person. The Apostle Paul, knowing this same law of contact and transmission that governed the operation of the Spirit of God in healing, laid his hands on cloths or handkerchiefs (Acts 19:11,12). Those cloths were taken to the sick, and the diseases departed from them.

Some people in modern times might think that the transfer of the anointing through cloth is only superstition. But it's not superstition; it's a viable fact. It happened just the way the Word of God said it happened.

In other words, the healing anointing, emanating from Paul, transformed those handkerchiefs into "storage batteries" of Holy Ghost power. When they were laid on the sick, they charged the body with the healing anointing, and the diseases departed from them.

Healing Anointing vs. Ministry Anointing

As I said at the beginning of this chapter, the anointing for ministry automatically comes with the calling to stand in whatever office God has called you to. But the *healing anointing* is something different and separate from a *ministry anointing*.

For instance, Jesus said to me when He appeared to me in the vision in Rockwall, Texas, in 1950: "I have called you before you were born. I separated you from your mother's womb. Satan tried to destroy your life before you were born and many times since then, but My angels have watched over you and cared for you until this present hour."

Well, when Jesus said, "I have called you," that didn't mean He called me on that very day, September 2, 1950. He had called me to the ministry before I was born. I understood what He meant when He said, "I have called you."

After Jesus said, "I have called you," He said, "and I have anointed you." Well, again, I knew He wasn't talking about anointing me for the ministry that very day. No, the anointing came with the calling, and I'd already been ministering with that anointing for many years.

But when Jesus said to me, "And I have given unto you a *special* anointing to lay hands on the sick," I knew He was talking about giving me a *special* anointing on that very day, September 2, 1950.

Now I had been laying hands on the sick for years and had seen them healed. But I wasn't ministering with a special anointing; I was just ministering to the sick through the laying on of hands according to the Word of God.

After Jesus gave me a special anointing in that vision to lay hands on the sick, He said to me, among other things, "This special anointing will not work for you unless you tell the people exactly what I've told you; that is, tell them you saw Me. Tell them I spoke to you, and that I laid the finger of My right hand in the palm of each of your hands. Tell them that the anointing is in your hands. Tell them exactly what I've told you. And tell them if they'll *believe* it—that you're anointed—and *receive* it, then that power will flow from your hands into their body, and will undo what Satan has wrought. It will effect a healing and a cure therein."

Now, the laying on of hands isn't the only way to minister, but it's one way. And it's a scriptural way.

Laying on of hands is a point of contact that releases the healing power. Sometimes the healing power of God is ministered to a sick person to the degree that he is manifestly charged with the power of God, just like a person might be charged with electricity. Yet no real or final healing takes place until something happens that releases the faith of the individual.

Healing Is by Degree

We need to understand that healing is by degree. And the degree of healing is determined by two conditions. Number one, *the degree of healing power administered to the body*. A person can be less anointed or more anointed to minister healing just like a preacher can be less anointed or more anointed to preach.

In the same way, a person can be less anointed or more anointed with the healing anointing. I've noticed that when the anointing upon me is manifested in a greater degree, we have more healings take place in the service.

The second condition that determines the degree of healing is *the degree of faith released by the individual to give action to that healing power*.

You can see this in Mark chapter 5, in the case with the woman with the issue of blood. Jesus said, *". . . Daughter, thy faith hath made thee whole . . . "* (v. 34). Someone might say, "I thought it was the power that flowed out of Jesus that made her whole." Yes, it was. *But it was her faith that gave action to that power.*

Jesus Christ and the Apostle Paul revealed and applied the laws that govern the operation of the healing anointing—the power of God. They demonstrated that the healing power of God is a tangible, transmittable, and measurable substance.

What was the power that flowed from Jesus' hands or was stored in His garments? Was it power that was inherent in Him as the Son of God? No. Acts 10:38 says, *". . . God anointed Jesus of Nazareth with the HOLY GHOST and POWER: who went about doing good, and healing all that were oppressed of the devil. . . ."*

Where did that power come from? It came from God. And that same power—the healing power of God—is available today.

Questions for Study

1. Any believer can lay hands on the sick according to what scripture?

   _____

   _____

2. Complete this sentence: Jesus had the anointing _____ measure.
   Members of the Body of Christ have the anointing _____ measure.

3. List the three characteristics of the anointing mentioned in this chapter.

   _____

   _____

4. What were the people seeking to touch in Matthew chapter 14?

   _____

   _____

5. Name two ways the anointing may be transferred.

   _____

   _____

6. In Acts 19:11 and 12, Paul laid his hands on cloths or handkerchiefs. What happened when those cloths were taken to the sick?

   _____

   _____

7. What is the laying on of hands?

   _____

   _____

8. Name the two conditions by which the degree of healing is determined.

   _____

   _____

9. In the case of the woman with the issue of blood, what was it that gave action to the healing power?

   _____

   _____

10. Where did the power that flowed from Jesus' hands or was stored in His garments come from?

   _____

   _____

Chapter 20

Healing in Relation to Words

The subject of healing in relation to words is very important because it will help you understand how to turn your faith loose in the area of healing. Although there are many scriptures that reveal how important our words are, we will study only some of them in this chapter.

Our main focus in this chapter is to understand how we are healed by hearing and speaking words. Before we study *healing* in relation to words, let's look at *salvation* in relation to words because the principle is the same.

Acts 11:14 says *"Who shall tell thee words, whereby thou and all thy house shall be saved."* This verse is from the passage of Scripture that relates how Cornelius and his household were saved. It implies that there are words a person must hear in order to be saved.

In Acts chapter 11, we learn that Peter was called to stand before the brethren in Jerusalem and explain why he was preaching to the Gentiles. In this passage, Peter relates the vision he saw and tells how he went down to Cornelius' house.

Once Peter arrived at Cornelius' house, Cornelius explained how he had seen an angel stand in his house and say "Send men to Joppa and inquire at the house of Simon the tanner for Simon Peter, who when he is come will *tell you words whereby you and all your house shall be saved"* (Acts 11:13,14).

Someone might say, "Why would Cornelius need to hear words in order to be saved? I thought we were saved by grace through faith."

Well, that is true. Ephesians 2:8 says, *"For by grace are ye saved through faith; and that not of yourselves: it is the gift of God."* But, how does "faith to be saved" come to us? It comes by hearing the Word of God (Rom 10:17). So we must hear the Word of God in order to have faith to be saved. And according to Romans 10:9 and 10, a person is not saved just by *hearing* the Word of God, but by also *speaking* the Word of God. In

other words, a person is saved by hearing and speaking words.

ROMANS 10:9,10
9 That if thou shalt confess with thy mouth the Lord Jesus, and shalt believe in thine heart that God hath raised him from the dead, thou shalt be saved.
10 For with the heart man believeth unto righteousness; and with the mouth confession is made unto salvation.

In Romans chapter 10, we see how men are *saved* by hearing and speaking words. By the same token, people are also *healed* by hearing and speaking words. You see, faith for healing comes the same way that faith for salvation comes, and that is by hearing the Word of God. And it is always with the heart that man believes and with the mouth that confession is made.

You see, you can have faith in Jesus, both as Lord and as Savior, but if you don't confess it as so in your life, it won't change anything. It won't come to fruition in your life. There's no such thing as a "secret believer." The Bible says that it is with the mouth that confession is made unto salvation (Rom. 10:10). And Matthew 10:32 says, *"Whosoever therefore shall confess me before men, him will I confess also before my Father which is in heaven."* It is very important to confess with your mouth what you believe in your heart.

Most Christians know this principle of believing with the heart and confessing with the mouth when it comes to salvation, or what we call the New Birth. But, this principle is also true when it comes to receiving anything from God. Healing is in the same plan of Redemption that the New Birth is. Just as we are saved by hearing and speaking words, so are we healed by hearing and speaking words.

Divine Intervention

Many Christians who desire healing are waiting for the intervention of divine sovereignty—for God to initiate something on His own. Of course, God does occasionally move in a sovereign way, but that is not His ordinary way of doing things. I'll show you in the Bible what I mean by the intervention of divine sovereignty, or God initiating something on His own.

JOHN 5:1-4
1 After this there was a feast of the Jews; and Jesus went up to Jerusalem.
2 Now there is at Jerusalem by the sheep market a pool, which is called in the Hebrew tongue Bethesda, having five porches.
3 In these lay a great multitude of impotent folk, of blind, halt, withered, waiting for the moving of the water.
4 For an angel went down at a certain season into the pool, and troubled the water: whosoever then first after the troubling of the water stepped in was made whole of whatsoever disease he had.

In this passage, we read that the first person who stepped into the pool of Bethesda after the angel had troubled the water was healed of whatever illness he had. It didn't make any difference what the illness was, and it didn't make any difference whether the sick person was an adult or a child, a man or a woman. It didn't make any difference whether they were God-fearing or not—or, as we would say, saved or unsaved. It didn't make any difference whether they were pretty or ugly, rich or poor. And it didn't make any difference what color their skin was. The first person in the pool got healed and was the only one to get healed. It was that simple.

In the case of the pool of Bethesda, God worked the healing miracles on His own. It's true that if God wants to work a miracle, He can. He doesn't have to ask me or you or anyone else permission to do so. And that's what is meant by the intervention of divine sovereignty or God initiating something on His own.

When God initiates something on His own and there is an intervention of divine sovereignty, very often only one person gets healed. Someone may ask, "Why?" Well, I don't know. If I knew, I could tell you why, but I'm not the one who is doing it! God is.

Jesus Calms the Storm

Mark chapter 4 gives us another example of divine intervention.

MARK 4:35-40
35 And the same day, when the even was come, he saith unto them, Let us pass over unto the other side.
36 And when they had sent away the multitude, they took him even as he was in the ship. And there were also with him other little ships.
37 And there arose a great storm of wind, and the waves beat into the ship, so that it was now full.
38 And he was in the hinder part of the ship, asleep on a pillow: and they awake him, and say unto him, Master, carest thou not that we perish?
39 And he arose, and rebuked the wind, and said unto the sea, Peace, be still. And the wind ceased, and there was a great calm.
40 And he said unto them, Why are ye so fearful? how is it that ye have no faith?

This miracle didn't happen on account of the disciples' faith, because in verse 40, Jesus asked His disciples why they didn't have any faith. Jesus expected them to have faith because He had told them, "Let us pass over to the other side" (v. 35). He hadn't said, "Let's go halfway and sink." No, this miracle didn't happen because the disciples had faith. The Lord just did it on His own.

God will do that sometimes. Unfortunately, many Christians are waiting for some kind of divine intervention to happen in their lives. It may happen, but it may not happen. But one thing I'm sure of: God's best, God's greatest, and everything God has is at our disposal by the claim of faith. We don't have to wait for His divine intervention, which may or may not happen. We don't have to wait for God to initiate something in a special way.

Walking on Water

We find another illustration of a divine intervention in Matthew chapter 14.

MATTHEW 14:25-31
25 And in the fourth watch of the night Jesus went unto them, walking on the sea.

26 And when the disciples saw him walking on the sea, they were troubled, saying, It is a spirit; and they cried out for fear.

27 But straightway Jesus spake unto them, saying, Be of good cheer; it is I; be not afraid.

28 And Peter answered him and said, Lord, if it be thou, bid me come unto thee on the water.

29 And he said, Come. And when Peter was come down out of the ship, he walked on the water, to go to Jesus.

30 But when he saw the wind boisterous, he was afraid; and beginning to sink, he cried, saying, Lord, save me.

31 And immediately Jesus stretched forth his hand, and caught him, and said unto him, O thou of little faith, wherefore didst thou doubt?

It wasn't Peter's faith that saved him. He had a little faith to walk on the water for a while, but then he started to sink. The Lord, through His own kindness and goodness, saved Peter.

There is something about God initiating something on His own that none of us can understand. There is a mystery about it. If we could understand everything about God, He would cease to be God. We don't even understand everything about humans, much less God. Why do we try to figure God out when we need to just accept Him as God? We ought to let Him tend to His business, and we should tend to ours.

Remember, in the case of the angel troubling the water in John chapter 5, only one person got healed. This is one example of God initiating something on His own in the area of healing. We've studied other examples of divine intervention including the time Jesus stilled the water and caused the storm to cease in Mark chapter 4 and the time He saved Peter from drowning in Matthew chapter 14. These two acts of sovereignty were in the area of saving people.

While God does occasionally intervene on His own initiative, we need to understand that it is not God's ordinary way of doing things. He ordinarily does things in our lives through our faith—by us believing Him and taking Him at His Word. The reason He has given us His Word is so that we can have faith, for we know that "faith comes by hearing and hearing by the Word of God" (Rom. 10:17).

Are You Waiting for God To Intervene?

Unfortunately, many Christians are waiting for divine intervention. They are waiting for God to initiate something out of the ordinary, which He may or He may not do, while all the time, God's best—everything He has for us—is at our disposal by the claim of faith.

I remember a dear lady who was bedfast with terminal cancer. Medical science did all they could do for her, and then they gave her up to die. This lady was not a member of the church where I was preaching, but the pastor had visited her and she told him that she wanted me to come and pray for her.

I went with the pastor to visit her. As always, I looked to the Lord to see if He would initiate or say something. He didn't say anything. I didn't have any kind of manifestation of the Spirit.

Well, what do you do if the Lord doesn't initiate something? You give people the Word of God. You put the Word into them in order to get them to believe God. And if you can get them to believe God, then you can agree with them.

So that's what I began to do with this lady who was dying of cancer. I began to give her the Word so that she could believe and be healed. But she wasn't interested in believing the Word of God. She was convinced that there was a person somewhere who was going to heal her.

I told her, "I'm sorry to disappoint you, sister, but there is no one anywhere who can heal *you* or anyone else. No person can do it."

She said, "Well, I'll just lie here and hope that there will be."

I said, "You will die in hope then."

And I'm sad to say that she did die.

Healing by a Manifestation of the Spirit

I knew another woman who was bedfast and dying with terminal cancer. She had deteriorated to the point where she couldn't even feed herself, much less get up out of bed. As we prayed together, there was a manifestation of the Spirit. In other words, the Lord initiated something.

Now, please understand this: I can't initiate a manifestation of the Spirit. I am not God. But, as I prayed for this woman, I heard the Lord speak to me and tell me to do something. So I did what He said to do; I went to the head of the bed and said, "Come out, you spirit of doubt and fear in the Name of Jesus."

The woman rose up shouting and jumped out of bed. She went from not being able to get out of bed to being instantly healed. She went out in the backyard and sat down and ate watermelon with us that very afternoon! Glory to God!

The Lord initiated something on His own that day. Now, I'd be a fool to tell everyone who has cancer that that's the way healing is ministered. I'd be a fool to tell people, "I found out how to get people healed. Just cast the spirit of doubt and fear out of every one of them." No, that may not be the problem with every person.

Again, if the Lord doesn't tell you anything, just put the Word into people. There is a connection between God's Word and healing. People are healed by hearing and saying words.

Healed by Hearing and Speaking God's Word

I knew another woman who had been diagnosed with terminal cancer and was told by her doctor that medical science had done all they could do for her. When I went to pray for her there wasn't any manifestation of the Spirit— the Spirit of God didn't say anything to me. What did I do? I did the same thing I tried to do with the first woman who was dying; I gave her the Word.

But unlike the first woman, this woman decided she would put God's Word into practice for herself. She received the Word as I gave it to her and began to speak it. And do you know what happened? The same doctors who diagnosed her couldn't find any cancer in her body—it had disappeared! She was healed by hearing and speaking God's Word!

Years later, I went back and preached in that woman's home church. Even then, the doctors still couldn't find anything wrong with her. When the cancer disappeared, the doctors told her that if it didn't reoccur after a certain number of years, she would be home free. And about the time I revisited her church, the doctors had told her, "That's it. You're home free. That cancer won't ever occur again."

Remember, I didn't lay hands on that woman and pray for her to be healed. It was *her faith* in God's Word that made her whole.

You see, all of God's provision is ours by the claim of faith. But faith must be released through the words of your mouth. Let me remind you of what Jesus said in Mark 11:23: *"For verily I say unto you, That whosoever shall SAY unto this mountain, Be thou removed, and be thou cast into the sea; and shall not doubt in his heart, but shall believe that those things which he SAITH shall come to pass; he shall have whatsoever he SAITH."* While doubt can cause you to receive something less than God's best, faith will cause you to receive God's best. And, remember, faith must be released through your words.

The Importance of Words

As I said at the beginning of the chapter, the Bible makes it clear that the words we speak are very important. Let's look at just a few verses that reveal the importance of our words.

Proverbs 18:21 says, *"Death and life are in the power of the tongue: and they that love it shall eat the fruit thereof."* Instead of saying, "death and life," you could say, "sickness and disease and healing and health are in the power of the tongue." Matthew 12:37, which says, *"For by thy words thou shalt be justified, and by thy words thou shalt be condemned,"* also shows the importance of our words.

Proverbs 21:23 says, *"Whoso keepeth his mouth and his tongue keepeth his soul from troubles."* This verse implies that we create our own troubles with our mouth and tongue. Many Christians think that someone else creates all their troubles. So these Christians are always complaining and blaming someone else for their problems, but this verse says that *they* created their own troubles.

Proverbs 12:18 says, *"There is that speaketh like the piercings of a sword: but the tongue of the wise is health."* The tongue of the wise is health because the tongue of the wise says the right things. You're going to produce either sickness or health with your tongue, mouth, and words. They all go together.

We need to understand that faith will cause the power of God to move in our behalf, and faith will cause us to receive the miraculous into our lives. But faith has to be released through the words of our mouth. Remember Mark 11:23 says, *". . . he shall have whatsoever he SAITH."* Faith is released through words. It's so with salvation, and it's so with healing.

Faith for salvation is released through the words of your mouth. We've already looked at Romans 10:9 and 10, which says, *"That if thou shalt confess with thy mouth the Lord Jesus, and shalt believe in thine heart that God hath raised him from the dead, thou shalt be saved. For with the heart man believeth unto righteousness; and with the mouth confession is made unto salvation."* With your heart you believe unto righteousness—you believe you are right with God because Jesus paid the price and made you right. And with your mouth confession is made unto salvation—with your mouth you confess that you are saved.

It works the same way with healing. With the heart man believes unto healing, and with the mouth he confesses he is healed. And even if a person gets healed by God initiating something on His own or by a manifestation of the gifts of the Spirit, he will not maintain that healing without maintaining a positive faith confession, because the devil will come and take it away. I've seen it happen again and again. We are healed by the words we speak, and we maintain our healing by the words we speak.

What Are You Saying?

Again, faith is released by words—whether it's faith to be saved, faith to be healed, or faith for any one of God's provisions. So it's important that you learn to use words so they will work

for you and not *against* you. We know from the Word of God that your words will either make you a victor or keep you a captive.

Words like these will make you a victor: "I am more than a conqueror through Him that loved me and gave Himself for me" (Rom. 8:37). "If God be for me, who can be against me?" (Rom. 8:31). "My Father is greater than all" (John 10:29). "The Name of Jesus has authority and power in Heaven, on earth, and under the earth—among angels, men, and demons. And that Name belongs to me" (Phil. 2:9,10; Matt. 28:18). Speaking the right words—God's Word—will set you free and keep you free.

But your words can also keep you captive. If you keep on talking about how you are defeated, saying, "Poor old me. I've tried and tried. Everything is against me. The devil keeps me sick all the time," things will stay just as they are or get worse.

You see, friends, if we're defeated, we're defeated with our own lips. People will lay their problems off on the devil or on someone else; sometimes they will even lay them off on the preacher. But we might as well get down to brass tacks, so to speak. If I'm defeated, I'm the one responsible. If you're defeated, you're the one responsible. Why? We are defeated with our own lips.

There is another verse in Proverbs having to do with words that has always been a favorite of mine. Proverbs 6:2 says, *"Thou art snared with the words of thy mouth, thou art taken with the words of thy mouth."* The margin of my *King James* Bible reads, "Thou art *taken captive* with the words of thy mouth."

Someone once said, "You said that you could not, and the moment you said it, you were whipped." I like to say it like this: "You said that you did not have faith, and doubt rose up like a giant and bound you." You see, you are imprisoned with your own words. If you talk failure, failure will hold you in bondage, for Proverbs 6:2 says, "You are snared with the words of your mouth."

As Christians, we should never talk failure or defeat. I don't know about you, but I don't believe in failure or defeat. And I don't believe that God is a God of failure or a God of defeat. Since we are children of God, we ought not be children of failure. I believe God is a God of victory and success, prosperity and plenty.

If you talk about your trials and difficulties or your lack of faith, your faith will shrivel, and the devil will rise up and dominate you. Confessing sickness will develop sickness in your system. Confessing doubt causes doubts to grow stronger. How well I have learned this truth through the years!

If you talk about your doubts and fears, it will destroy your faith. But if you reverse what you are talking about, it will change the order of things. What should you talk about then? You ought to talk about your wonderful, lovely Heavenly Father. You should talk about the Word of God. But, you see, if you don't know God, you won't be able to talk about Him. You need to get acquainted with God through His Word and through prayer. God is everything the Word says He is, and He can do everything the Word says He can do. So find out what the Word says!

Spend your time talking about who God is and what He can do. Then look defeat in the face and cry out, "My God is greater than you!" Look failure in the face and declare, "My God is greater than you!"

Remember, you can't be defeated because greater is He that is in you than he that's in the world (1 John 4:4). God is greater than sickness and disease. He is greater than troubles and trials. He's greater than any power that can come against you. You can't measure how great God is!

Begin talking about your wonderful Heavenly Father. Begin saying, "God is everything the Word says He is. God can do everything the Words says He can do." Start talking about how big God is, and quit talking about how big the devil is. What does the devil amount to in the sight of God? Nothing! Jesus already whipped him! Start talking about that!

When you read God's Word, believe it, and begin to confess it. Remember, your words are important. Use them to work *for* you as you receive by faith everything God has provided for you—including healing!

Questions for Study

1. What does Acts 11:14 imply?

2. How does faith to be saved come to us?

3. How does faith for healing come?

4. What are many Christians who desire healing waiting for?

5. In the case of the angel troubling the water in John chapter 5, how many people got healed?

6. How does God ordinarily do things in our lives?

7. How is all of God's provision yours?

8. How must faith be released?

9. Why is the tongue of the wise health?

10. What will cause the power of God to move in our behalf and cause us to receive the miraculous into our lives?

Chapter 21

God's Great Mercy—Part 1

The Lord is gracious, and full of compassion; slow to anger, and of great mercy. The Lord is good to all: and his tender mercies are over all his works.

—Psalm 145:8,9

Nothing reveals the character of God more than these two verses of Scripture. The Lord is gracious! *And* He's full of compassion. The dictionary tells us that "to be full of compassion" means *to be merciful*. So "compassion" and "mercy" are companion terms, we might say.

And, if you look up the words "compassion" and "mercy," you'll find that often the same Hebrew or Greek word is translated one time "mercy" and another time "compassion."

Therefore, "to have mercy" means *to be full of compassion*. God is full of compassion, He is of great mercy, and His tender mercies are over all of His works.

I want to talk to you about the subject of mercy. It's such a big subject that I can't cover it all in one chapter, but I want to emphasize one certain part of it. Usually we think of "mercy" only in connection with the Lord having mercy on the sinner and saving him. Well, that's a part of it, but we also need to think of God's mercy in connection with healing.

The first text we will look at is in Mark chapter 1. I want you to notice some things about the Lord Jesus Christ. Because Jesus is the will of God in action, we can look at God's compassion manifested in the Person of Jesus.

MARK 1:40-42
**40 And there came a leper to him, beseeching him, and kneeling down to him, and saying unto him, If thou wilt, thou canst make me clean.
41 And Jesus, moved with compassion, put forth his hand, and touched him, and saith unto him, I will; be thou clean.**

42 And as soon as he had spoken, immediately the leprosy departed from him, and he was cleansed.

Notice that compassion moved Jesus to heal the leper. Healing is a display of God's compassion.

Compassion Compelled Jesus

Let's look at another example of the Lord's compassion in relation to healing.

MATTHEW 14:13,14
**13 . . . [Jesus] departed thence by ship into a desert place apart: and when the people had heard thereof, they followed him on foot out of the cities.
14 And Jesus went forth, and saw a great multitude, and was moved with compassion toward them, and he healed their sick.**

Verse 14 says that Jesus was moved with compassion. Well, what did compassion move Him to do? It moved Him to heal! Verse 14 says, *". . . and he [Jesus] healed their sick."*

I think that the compassion of the Lord in connection with healing has been hidden from us because it has been taught that Jesus healed the sick only to prove His deity. Yet that kind of statement isn't in the Bible. Not once, in all the recorded cases of healing, does the Bible ever say, ". . . and to prove His deity and divinity, Jesus healed them." And if the Bible doesn't say it, then we shouldn't say it either.

According to the Bible, Jesus healed the sick because of His compassion, not because of His deity or divinity. His compassion compelled Him to do it. And, thank God, He's the same compassionate Lord today.

God never changes. He's the same now as He was back then. So if He was gracious then, He's gracious now. If He was full of compassion then, He's full of compassion now. If He was merciful then, He's merciful now.

Healing Is a Mercy

The third example of God's great mercy manifested in the Person of Jesus Christ in the area of healing is in Matthew chapter 20.

MATTHEW 20:29-34
29 And as they departed from Jericho, a great multitude followed him.
30 And, behold, two blind men sitting by the way side, when they heard that Jesus passed by, cried out, saying, Have mercy on us, O Lord, thou Son of David.
31 And the multitude rebuked them, because they should hold their peace: but they cried the more, saying, Have mercy on us, O Lord, thou Son of David.
32 And Jesus stood still, and called them, and said, What will ye that I shall do unto you?
33 They say unto him, Lord, that our eyes may be opened.
34 So Jesus had compassion on them, and touched their eyes: and immediately their eyes received sight, and they followed him.

The two blind men in this passage cried out for Jesus to have mercy on them. When Jesus asked these men what they wanted, they did not say, "That our sins may be forgiven." You see, we usually think of mercy in connection with the forgiveness or remission of sins. We think of the mercy of God extended toward the sinner. But is He any less merciful to the sick? These men were asking for mercy in connection with healing.

If they had asked for their sins to be forgiven, that would be mercy all right. But when Jesus asked them what they wanted, they answered, "That we might receive our sight." Healing is a mercy, too.

Verse 34 says that Jesus had compassion—or mercy—on them and "*. . . touched their eyes: and immediately their eyes received sight, and they followed him.*"

Now, let's review what happened in this passage. These two blind men asked for the mercy of having their eyes opened. Jesus granted unto them the mercy of healing, *proving* that healing is a mercy just as forgiveness is a mercy.

The Father of Mercies

Mercy isn't just something that God has or shows; it's part of His nature.

2 CORINTHIANS 1:3
3 Blessed be God, even the Father of our Lord Jesus Christ, the FATHER OF MERCIES, and the God of all comfort.

This verse of Scripture reveals the character of my Father God. So many times we as Christians don't see God our Father in the light that we should. As I've said many times before, some Christians picture God as a sort of traffic cop who is just waiting for them to do something wrong so He can blow the whistle on them. Or they picture God as an austere judge who is waiting, with gavel in hand, to smite them the minute they do wrong. Or they picture God as waiting with a giant flyswatter, ready to swat them as soon as they stop moving.

Yes, God is against wrongdoing, and He is a God of justice. But Second Corinthians 1:3 tells us that He is also the Father of mercies.

'Guilty, Your Honor'

I remember holding a meeting in a particular Full Gospel Church and traveling to the meeting one night with a gentleman who I had asked to be a special singer. One night while we were driving to the revival meeting that was some distance away, he began telling me a story about something that had happened to him recently.

This was back in the Depression days, and this man owned a little business. He was what we call a "lay preacher" because he was never in full-time ministry. Usually, this man would sing in meetings, but sometimes pastors would ask him to preach if they had to be gone from the church.

A pastor contacted this man because an emergency arose and asked him to take care of the Wednesday night service. And so this gentleman said he would do it.

Well, back in Depression days, places of business didn't operate for just eight hours. This man's business was open nearly every hour it could possibly be open. So on the day the pastor asked him to take the service, this man was busy working. He didn't have time to do a lot of praying or studying for that night's service.

As this man left for the service, he realized he was running late and was going to have to rush in order to make it on time. He had to drive through two or three little towns to get to the church. And while he was driving, he tried to meditate on scriptures for that night's message.

One of the small towns he drove through didn't have but two red lights in the whole town. Preoccupied with preparing for the service, he ran one of them. About that time, he heard a siren and looked up to see flashing red lights right behind him.

He pulled over, and the policeman came up to him and said, "Do you realize what you did? You not only ran a red light, but you were also driving thirty miles an hour in a twenty-five mile an hour zone."

The man answered, "Well, Officer, if you say so, then it must have been so. I didn't even know there was a red light back there. I'll be honest with you. I was on my way to preach, and I should have been paying attention, but I wasn't. I'm in the wrong; that's all there is to it. Go ahead, and write me a ticket."

The officer said, "Well, you did run the red light and break the speed limit, but I'm just going to give you a ticket for speeding. We'll forget about the other."

Well, this man didn't have the money to pay for the ticket, so he had to appear before the local judge who would decide what he would have to do to work off what he owed.

When he stood before the judge, the judge asked, "How do you plead?"

He answered, "Sir, I'm guilty if this young man [the policeman] says so." And then he went on to explain the situation to the judge exactly how he had explained it to the policeman.

The judge said, "Just because you were going to a service and so forth is no excuse."

The man replied, "Judge, I don't have the money to pay the ticket. You'll just have to put me in jail. That's all there is to it."

(In those days they had what they called the "county farm" or the "pea patch." And anyone who couldn't pay his fine was required to work on the county farm in order to pay it off.)

Justice or Mercy?

Then the man went on to say, "Judge, I didn't come here to plead for justice; I don't need that, because if I get justice I'm going to jail. I came here to plead for mercy."

Then he added, "Sir, I don't know whether or not you're a Christian."

The Judge said, "Yes, I am. I teach a Bible class at Such-and-such church."

The man continued, "Well, then you ought to know the Bible. Do you remember the story in John chapter 8 about the woman who was caught in adultery? Under the law she was supposed to be stoned to death. As the people prepared to stone her, they asked Jesus about the law. He answered them by saying, 'Let him who is without sin cast the first stone' (v. 7). Then Jesus stooped down and wrote something in the sand. When He looked up, everyone was gone. He said, 'Woman, where are your accusers?' She said, 'I have none.' So Jesus said, 'Neither do I condemn you. Go and sin no more.'

The man continued, "Now, I did wrong all right, but if you'll have mercy upon me, I'll promise you I won't do that anymore. I'll go and sin no more."

The judge replied, "You mean that story is in the Bible?"

The man happened to have his New Testament with him, so he opened it to John chapter 8 and showed it to the judge. The judge read the passage and said, "Case dismissed." And then he added, "I'm going to teach that to my Sunday school class next Sunday."

This man asked the judge for mercy because that's what he needed. He didn't need justice; he needed mercy.

'Mercies' Is Plural!

Isn't it good to know that God is the Father of mercies? Yes, He is a God of justice, but He is also the Father of mercies. If He wasn't, none of us would be alive today.

Let's take a closer look at Second Corinthians 1:3.

2 CORINTHIANS 1:3
3 Blessed be God, even the Father of our Lord Jesus Christ, the FATHER OF MERCIES, and the God of all comfort.

Notice this verse doesn't say that God is the Father of *mercy*, singular. It says He is the Father of *mercies*, plural! You see, if He was just the Father of one mercy—the mercy of forgiveness toward the sinner, for example—then Paul would have called Him the Father of mercy. But, thank God, He's the Father of mercies, and one of His mercies is healing!

Telling of the Lord's Compassion

In Mark chapter 5, we read that Jesus delivered a man possessed by a devil. I want to call your attention to the fact that Jesus had compassion on this man who was possessed by a devil, who broke the chains that bound him, and who wandered among the tombs, crying out day and night while cutting himself with stones. Jesus had compassion upon this man, and the man was delivered, healed, clothed, and restored to his right mind.

We know that Jesus healed him out of compassion, because Mark 5:19 says, *"Howbeit Jesus suffered him not, but saith unto him, Go home to thy friends, and tell them how great things the Lord hath done for thee, and hath had compassion on thee."* This verse implies that the Lord did great things for the man because the Lord had compassion on him.

The man did just as Jesus told him to do. Mark 5:20 says, *"And he [the man] departed, and began to publish in Decapolis how great things Jesus had done for him: and all men did marvel."* And because this man told others about the Lord's compassion (Jesus told him to "tell what things the Lord has done for you and how He had compassion on you."), multitudes came to Jesus to be healed. How do we know that? Matthew chapter 15 tells us so.

MATTHEW 15:30,31
30 And great multitudes came unto him [Jesus], having with them those that were lame, blind, dumb, maimed, and many others, and cast them down at Jesus' feet; and he healed them:
31 Insomuch that the multitude wondered, when they saw the dumb to speak, the maimed to be whole, the lame to walk, and the blind to see: and they glorified the God of Israel.

Now it's important for us to realize that the setting of this passage is Decapolis—the same place the man in Mark chapter 5 was to go and tell about the Lord's compassion. You may not realize that it is the same place without a close study of the Word, but it is (*see* Mark 7:31-37 for the parallel account of Matthew 15:30 and 31).

As a result of this man publishing, or telling about, the Lord's compassion, great multitudes came to Jesus and were healed. Again the Word says, *"And great multitudes came unto him [Jesus], having with them those that were lame, blind, dumb, maimed, and many others, and cast them down at Jesus' feet; and he healed them: Insomuch that the multitude wondered, when they saw the dumb to speak, the maimed to be whole, the lame to walk, and the blind to see: and they glorified the God of Israel"* (Matt. 15:30,31). All those healings came about because of the testimony of this one man, because he published, or told about, the Lord's compassion.

Is God Still Merciful?

Some people say healing isn't for us today. Well, is *compassion* for us today? Of course, it is! And is the Lord still compassionate and merciful? Of course, He is! We have seen in the New Testament that the words "compassion" and "mercy" are consistently mentioned in connection with healing. So we know that because God's mercy is still for us today, *healing* is also for us today!

Remember, God is the Father of *mercies*. Not only is the forgiveness of sin and the remission of sin a mercy, but *healing* is a mercy! If you will simply think of healing as one of God's tender mercies, you'll find right away that you'll get somewhere.

God is merciful to save, and He is merciful to heal. Thank God for the mercy of healing!

Questions for Study

1. What does "to have mercy" mean?

   _____

   _____

2. What do we usually think of mercy in connection with?

   _____

   _____

3. What moved Jesus to heal the leper in Mark chapter 1?

   _____

   _____

4. Complete this sentence: According to the Bible, Jesus healed the sick because of His _____, not because of His _____ or _____.

5. When Jesus asked the blind men in Matthew chapter 20 what they wanted, what did they answer?

   _____

   _____

6. Complete this sentence: Mercy isn't just something that God has or shows; it's _____ _____ _____ _____.

7. God is a God of justice, but what is He the Father of?

   _____

   _____

8. Because of what Scripture verse do we know that Jesus healed the devil-possessed man because of compassion?

   _____

   _____

9. After the devil-possessed man was healed, what happened as a result of him publishing, or telling about, the Lord's compassion?

   _____

   _____

10. Complete this sentence: Because God's _____ is still for us today, _____ is also for us today.

Chapter 22

God's Great Mercy—Part 2

In the last chapter, we began studying God's great mercy. We read several New Testament examples of how Jesus displayed mercy during His ministry on the earth. In this chapter, we are going to show that God's mercy hasn't been modified since Jesus' ascension but rather is still being manifested in Jesus' present-day ministry as our faithful High Priest.

The first text I want to look at is John 16:7.

JOHN 16:7
7 Nevertheless I [Jesus] tell you the truth; It is expedient for you that I go away: for if I go not away, the Comforter will not come unto you; but if I depart, I will send him unto you.

The word "expedient" in this verse means *profitable*. So in other words, Jesus told His disciples, "It's *profitable* for you that I go away." That means Jesus thought it was a good thing that He go to Heaven and the Holy Ghost or Comforter be given unto man. In his book *Christ the Healer*, F. F. Bosworth points out that Jesus' going away could not be profitable (and thus Jesus' statement proved untrue) "if His going away would withdraw, or even modify, the manifestation of His compassion in healing the sick."[1]

Brother Bosworth went on to say, "Every man who teaches that healing is not for all who need it today, as it was in the past, is virtually teaching that Christ's compassion toward the sick has been at least modified since His exaltation. Worse yet, others teach that [Jesus'] compassion in healing the sick has been entirely withdrawn. To me, it is a mystery how any minister can take a position that veils and interferes with the manifestation of the greatest attribute of deity, God's compassion which is Divine Love in action."[2]

Jesus Is the Same Yesterday, Today, and Forever

Why would Jesus be any less compassionate in His present-day ministry as our faithful High Priest than He was in His earthly ministry? Jesus is the same now as He was when He was on the earth. He never changes. He's the same now as He was back then. So if He was gracious then, He's gracious now. If He was full of compassion then, He's full of compassion now. If He was merciful then, He's merciful now.

HEBREWS 2:17
17 Wherefore in all things it behoved him to be made like unto his brethren, that he might be a MERCIFUL and faithful high priest in things pertaining to God, to make reconciliation for the sins of the people.

The same Greek word translated "merciful" in this verse is also translated "compassionate" in other passages. We've already brought out the fact that both the words "merciful" and "compassionate" can be used interchangeably. Therefore, the Greek adjective translated "merciful" in Hebrews 4:17 could also be translated "compassionate." Both of these words accurately describe Jesus our High Priest.

Hebrews 4:15 tells us that Jesus our High Priest understands what we're going through and has compassion on us.

HEBREWS 4:15
15 For we have not an high priest which cannot be TOUCHED with the feeling of our infirmities; but was in all points tempted like as we are, yet without sin.

We know that this verse refers to the compassion of Jesus because the same Greek word translated "touched" here in verse 15 is translated "have compassion" in Hebrews 10:34, which says, *"For ye had COMPASSION of me in my bonds, and took joyfully the spoiling of your goods, knowing in yourselves that ye have in heaven a better and an enduring substance."* You see, Jesus is touched with, or has compassion for, the feeling of our infirmities. He's no less compassionate now than He was two thousand years ago.

So if Jesus is the same today as He was yesterday—if He is the same now as our exalted High Priest sitting at the right hand of the Father as He was when He walked the shores of Galilee—then He is full of just as much compassion now as He was then. That means Jesus is full of just as much compassion and mercy today as He was in Matthew chapter 20 when He departed from Jericho and two blind men cried unto Him, "Have mercy on us, thou Son of David." He stopped and asked them, "What will you that I do unto you?" They said, "That we might receive our sight." And Jesus had compassion, or mercy, on them and healed them (Matt. 20:29-34).

If Jesus is the same now as He was then, then He's still full of compassion. And the Bible tells us that He *is* the same now as He was when He was on the earth (Heb. 13:8). When you can get people to see that, getting them healed is no problem at all.

The Lord Wants You Healed

Very often I tell people who want healing that the Lord wants to heal them even more than they want to be healed. Most of them look at me in astonishment when I say that. I tell them, "He wants you to be well more than you want to be well. He *yearns* to heal you."

I have asked individual people, "Do you believe in divine healing?"

And I've had born-again, Spirit-filled people answer, "Oh, yes. My church believes in divine healing."

I tell them, "Just because your church believes in divine healing doesn't mean you're going to get healed."

So they reply, "Yes, sir. I believe in divine healing."

But then when I tell them that God wants to heal them even more than they want to be healed, some of them, without even thinking, blurt out, "Oh, I wish I could believe that."

People who are *wishing that they could believe* that the Lord wants to heal them, don't really *know* that the Lord wants to heal them. Well, how can I get them to see that God does want to heal them? There is only one way, and that is to just keep giving them the Word of God.

During the many years I've been in ministry, I've had to give people the Word of God again and again. Some people I prayed for told me to leave them alone. I just said, "No, I'm not going to leave you alone," and then I'd hold them against the Word. In other words, I kept telling them what God's Word says about healing, and after a while, it registered in their hearts.

Compassion in Jesus' Present-Day Ministry

Because of the Lord's compassion and mercy, He *wants* to heal you. Just because Jesus has been exalted doesn't mean He's lost or modified His mercy. The Bible doesn't teach that His mercy has been done away with or modified. Rather, the Bible teaches that God's mercy has been increased. John 14:12 says, *"Verily, verily, I say unto you, He that believeth on me, the works that I do shall he do also; and GREATER WORKS than these shall he do; because I go unto my Father."*

Peter's Shadow

Acts chapter 5 gives us an example of Jesus' compassion being displayed in His present-day ministry. It's another wonderful proof of Christ's compassion toward the sick and another proof that He is the same now as He was when He was on the earth.

ACTS 5:15,16
15 Insomuch that they brought forth the sick into the streets, and laid them on beds and couches, that at the least the shadow of Peter passing by might overshadow some of them.
16 There came also a multitude out of the cities round about unto Jerusalem, bringing sick folks, and them which were vexed with unclean spirits: and they were healed every one.

Many Christians miss it here because they say, "Well, yes, that happened, but Peter did that." No, Peter didn't heal those people. And Peter's shadow didn't heal them either. It was Jesus, full of compassion, who healed them. Sometimes, our thinking is so limited that we get our eyes on people. Remember Jesus is the Head of the Church (Eph. 5:23; Col. 1:18), and He is the Healer!

God Wrought Special Miracles

In Acts chapter 19, we find an example of the Lord's compassion being displayed in the ministry of the Apostle Paul.

ACTS 19:11,12
11 And God wrought special miracles by the hands of Paul:
12 So that from his body were brought unto the sick handkerchiefs or aprons, and the diseases departed from them, and the evil spirits went out of them.

Who healed the sick in this passage? Was it Paul? No, it doesn't say, "Paul wrought special miracles by the hands of God." Verse 11 says, *". . . GOD wrought special miracles by the hands of Paul."* It was God who healed the sick. If we're not careful, we can get our eyes on man and think that man works the miracles.

Someone might say, "The handkerchiefs are what caused the miracle."

No, the handkerchiefs themselves didn't work the miracle. If that were the case, then any handkerchief could do it. No, God has to be involved.

Likewise, if it was just Peter's shadow in and of itself that healed the people, then years later, people would have still been getting healed by being in his shadow. But we don't see that happening. It was God who healed the people! He simply chose to do it through Peter's shadow. The Lord wanted to help the people so badly that He wrought special miracles as a display of His compassion and mercy.

The Lord's Compassion Is Manifested Through Believers

In Acts chapter 28, we find the Lord's compassion manifested again through Paul in the healing of all the people on the island of Melita.

ACTS 28:8,9
8   And it came to pass, that the father of Publius lay sick of a fever and of a bloody flux: to whom Paul entered in, and prayed, and laid his hands on him, and healed him.
9   So when this was done, others also, which had diseases in the island, came, and were healed.

Publius' father was healed after Paul laid hands on him, but it wasn't Paul who healed him. It was God. The man wasn't healed because Paul was a mighty apostle or because of any human ingenuity from a natural standpoint. Paul didn't minister to those people just as Paul the man or the apostle. He ministered to them empowered by the Holy Ghost and directed by the Lord Jesus Christ—the Head of the Church.

Notice that Paul entered in, prayed, and laid his hands on the sick man, and the man was healed. Why did Paul pray and lay hands on the man? Do you think he just thought that up himself? No. Remember what Jesus, the Head of the Church, said: *"And these signs shall follow them that believe; In my name . . . they shall lay hands on the sick, and they shall recover"* (Mark 16:17,18).

The Lord is still healing through His Name and through His followers. Are you going to do the greater works Jesus spoke of in John 14:12 because of your natural abilities? No, you will do the greater works because of Jesus and because He went unto His Father.

God Has More Than One Tender Mercy

We studied Psalm 145:8 and 9 in the previous chapter, and I want to look at it again in depth. In the light of all that we've studied, I think these verses will take on new meaning or will become more meaningful to you.

PSALM 145:8,9
8   The Lord is gracious, and full of compassion; slow to anger, and of great mercy.
9   The Lord is good to all: and his tender mercies are over all his works.

Think about that last phrase for a moment: "His tender mercies are over all His works." Were His tender mercies over His works of healing the sick? Yes, they were! The Bible tells us that Jesus was "moved with compassion" for the leper and healed him (Mark 1:40-42). We also read in the Bible that when Jesus saw the multitudes, He had compassion on them and healed their sick (Matt. 14:13,14). We know that "mercy" is another word for "compassion." His tender mercies are over all His works!

It is time to start believing in the Lord's mercy of healing. You probably don't have any problem at all believing in God's mercy of forgiveness because you've heard the message of forgiveness preached all your life. And you probably don't have any problem at all believing in God's mercy toward the sinner. If a sinner came to the altar and you were praying with him and he said, "Well, I don't know whether the Lord will save me or not," you'd be quick to tell him that the Lord would certainly forgive him. You might give him scripture after scripture about the Lord's mercy.

But, you see, that's as far as our thinking goes. We need to expand our thinking. We need to think God's thoughts after Him. How are you going to think God's thoughts? Think in line with what the Word says.

Someone may ask, "Is the mercy of healing available to me?" Well, is God's mercy of forgiveness available to the sinner? Yes, thank God. Is His mercy of forgiveness available to the Christian who has sinned or failed? Yes, thank God. But God's mercy doesn't stop there; His tender mercies are over *all* His works.

Well, we can thank God for the remission of sins and the New Birth. But that's not *all* His works. Notice again that Psalm 145:9 says "tender *mercies*," which is plural. The word "mercy" in this verse has to be plural because the verse says that God's mercies are over all His "works" which is plural. God's *works* are plural, and His *mercies* are plural.

Where does His mercy reach us? It reaches us in the spiritual realm, and it also reaches us in the natural realm. And, thank God, it reaches us in the financial and material realm. Because of God's mercies, not because of justice or because

we deserved anything, we are blessed in every area of our lives.

The Lord Is Good to *All*!

Let's read Psalm 145:8 and 9 again and study it phrase by phrase.

PSALM 145:8,9
8   The Lord is gracious, and full of compassion; slow to anger, and of great mercy.
9   The Lord is good to all: and his tender mercies are over all his works.

Psalm 145:8 says that the Lord is gracious and *full of compassion*. When I think of something being full, I automatically think about a glass being full of water. When a glass is full of water, then there isn't room for anything else. Well, the Lord is *full of compassion*!

Verse 8 also says that the Lord is slow to anger. I'm glad that He is! And I like the next phrase too: "He is of great mercy." If it just said that God was merciful, that would have been good, but this verse says that God is of *great* mercy!

Psalm 145:9 says, *"The Lord is good to ALL."* "All" means *everyone*! I've heard Christians say, "The Lord's been better to So-and-so than He's been to me." As a matter of fact, in times past, I've actually told the Lord, "You were better to So-and-so than You were to me."

You might ask, "Were you saved?" Yes, I wouldn't have been talking to Him if I hadn't been. Then you might ask, "What did He say to you?" Nothing. He just let me gripe and complain and fuss until I repented, and then He talked to me.

It would be funny if it weren't so pathetic. I've heard some people say, "Well, it looks like the Lord is better to everyone else than He is to me." And I've heard other people say, "The Lord is good to some people and bad to others."

People who say these kinds of things haven't experienced God's goodness for themselves, not because God isn't good to them, but because they haven't *received* His goodness. Even in the natural, there are some people who won't let you be good to them. Have you ever tried to be kind to someone, and they wouldn't receive it? Well, people can also reject God's goodness.

Again, Psalm 145:9 says, "The Lord is good to all." Now, we might think about someone as being a good person and say, "He's a good man," or "She's a good girl," or "So-and-so is a good person." Although God is good in the sense that we might say a person is good, that's not what this verse is saying. This verse is talking about God's goodness or His compassion toward us.

Naturally speaking, it's easy to be good to some people. But then there are others who make it difficult to be good to them. But, God is good to *all*!

Notice that "good to all" is in connection with the Lord being gracious and full of compassion. If God is good to all, then His compassion and mercy are available to all. In other words, God has made the same provision for every single one of us.

We know that God has made the same provision for everyone in the area of forgiveness of sins. No one doubts He has made the same provision for us in connection with the remission of sins. But, in His goodness and mercy, God has also made the same provision for us in the area of healing.

Matthew 8:17 says, "*. . . Himself* [Jesus] *took OUR infirmities, and bare OUR sicknesses.*" Who is the "our" in the verse referring to? All of us! And that includes *you!*

---

[1]F.F. Bosworth, *Christ the Healer*, (Michigan: Fleming H. Revell, 1973), p. 73.

[2]F.F. Bosworth, *Christ the Healer*, (Michigan: Fleming H. Revell, 1973), p. 74.

Questions for Study

1. Complete this sentence: God's mercy hasn't been _____ since Jesus' _____, but rather, it is still being _____ in Jesus' present-day ministry as our faithful _____ _____.

2. What does the word "expedient" mean?

    _____

    _____

3. How can the Greek word translated "merciful" also be translated?

    _____

    _____

4. Complete this sentence: People who are _____ that they could believe that the Lord wants to heal them don't really _____ that the Lord wants to heal them.

5. Because of the Lord's compassion and mercy, what does He want to do?

    _____

    _____

6. Give an example of Jesus' compassion being displayed through Peter's ministry.

    _____

    _____

7. Give an example of Jesus' compassion being displayed through Paul's ministry.

    _____

    _____

8. Complete this sentence: God's _____ are plural, and His _____ are plural.

9. Where does God's mercy reach us?

    _____

    _____

10. According to Psalm 145:9, how many people is the Lord good to?

    _____

    _____

STUDY GUIDES AVAILABLE

BY KENNETH E. HAGIN

Baptism in the Holy Spirit

This important study guide, which focuses on the baptism in the Holy Spirit and speaking in other tongues, teaches believers how to draw from the ever present source of power within them—the Holy Spirit.

Item No. BM063
ISBN-10: 0-89276-063-X / ISBN-13: 978-0-89276-063-3
Saddle bound—5.5" x 8.5"/ 66 pages

Biblical Ways to Receive Healing

There is no set way by which people may receive healing. And in this new study guide, you will discover various methods for receiving healing as recorded in the Word of God.

Item No. BM074
ISBN-10: 0-89276-074-5 / ISBN-13: 978-0-89276-074-9
Saddle bound—5.5" x 8.5"/ 71 pages

Foundations for Faith

Faith makes the difference between defeat and victory in a Christian's life. And this study guide explains why receiving from God is dependent upon the faith of the believer.

Item No. BM067
ISBN-10: 0-89276-067-2 / ISBN-13: 978-0-89276-067-1
Saddle bound—5.5" x 8.5"/ 64 pages

Gifts of the Holy Spirit

The lessons in this valuable study guide closely examine the gifts of the Holy Spirit, their operations, and their practical uses.

Item No. BM064
ISBN-10: 0-89276-064-8 / ISBN-13: 978-0-89276-064-0
Saddle bound—5.5" x 8.5" / 69 pages

God's Word on Divine Healing

This dynamic study guide gives convincing scriptural proof that it is God's will to heal!

Item No. BM069
ISBN-10: 0-89276-069-9 / ISBN-13: 978-0-89276-069-5
Saddle bound—5.5" x 8.5" / 77 pages

The Ministry Gifts

This informative, in-depth study guide discusses the biblical characteristics of the ministry gifts—apostle, prophet, evangelist, pastor, teacher—and their roles in the Body of Christ.

Item No. BM073
ISBN-10: 0-89276-073-7 / ISBN-13: 978-0-89276-073-2
Saddle bound—5.5" x 8.5" / 120 pages

Steps to Answered Prayer

Steps to Answered Prayer reveals step-by-step guidelines that, when faithfully followed in prayer, assure the believer of an answer.

Item No. BM065
ISBN-10: 0-89276-065-6
ISBN-13: 978-0-89276-065-7
Saddle bound—5.5" x 8.5" / 67 pages

Walking by Faith

Each lesson in this comprehensive study guide will help the believer achieve a workable operation of faith in his life—a faith that works.

Item No. BM068
ISBN-10: 0-89276-068-0
ISBN-13: 978-0-89276-068-8
Saddle bound—5.5" x 8.5"/ 67 pages

The Will of God in Prayer

This study guide will instruct believers on how to use the Word of God in prayer and get results.

Item No. BM066
ISBN-10: 0-89276-066-4
ISBN-13: 978-0-89276-066-4
Saddle bound—5.5" x 8.5" / 64 pages

"What should I do with my life?"

If you've been asking yourself this question, **RHEMA BIBLE TRAINING COLLEGE**

is a good place to come and find out. RBTC will build a solid biblical foundation

in you that will carry you through—wherever life takes you.

The Benefits:

◆ Training at *the* **top Spirit-filled Bible school**

◆ Teaching based on steadfast faith in God's Word

◆ Unique two-year core program specially designed to **grow** you as a believer, help you **recognize the voice of God**, and equip you to **live successfully**

◆ Optional **specialized training** in the third- and fourth-year program of your choice: Biblical Studies, Helps Ministry, Itinerant Ministry, Pastoral Ministry, Student Ministries, Worship, World Missions, and General Extended Studies

◆ **Accredited** with Transworld Accrediting Commission International

◆ Worldwide **ministry opportunities**— while you're in school

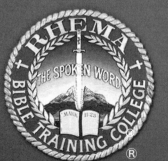

Apply today!

1-888-28-FAITH (1-888-283-2484)

rbtc.org

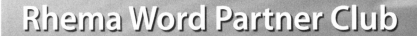
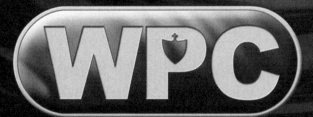

Always on.

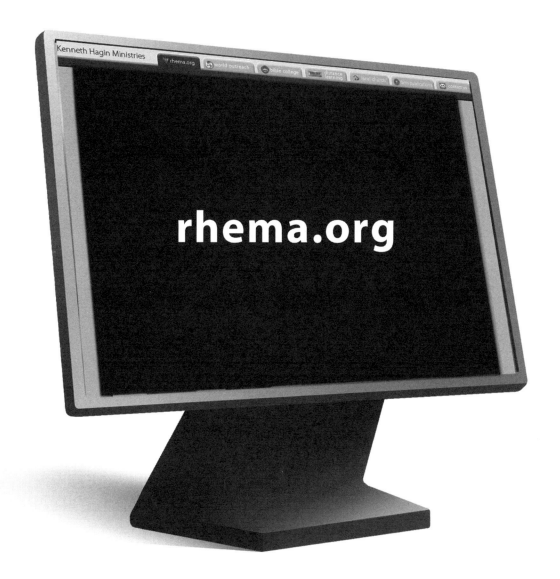

For the latest news and information on products, media, podcasts, study resources, and special offers, visit us online 24 hours a day.

rhema.org

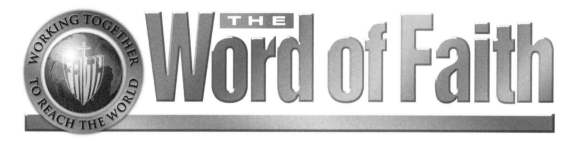

Free Subscription!

Call now to receive a free subscription to *The Word of Faith* magazine from Kenneth Hagin Ministries. Receive encouragement and spiritual refreshment from . . .

- *Faith-building articles from Kenneth W. Hagin, Lynette Hagin, Craig W. Hagin, and others*

- *"Timeless Teaching" from the archives of Kenneth E. Hagin*

- *Feature articles on prayer and healing*

- *Testimonies of salvation, healing, and deliverance*

- *Children's activity page*

- *Updates on Rhema Bible Training College, Rhema Bible Church, and other outreaches of Kenneth Hagin Ministries*

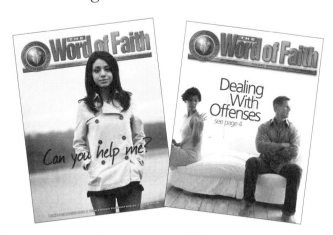

Subscribe today for your free *Word of Faith*!

1-888-28-FAITH (1-888-283-2484)

rhema.org/wof

Notes:

Notes:

Notes:

Notes:

Notes:

Notes: